Laughing and Loving with Autism

A collection of "real life" warm
and humorous stories

R. Wayne Gilpin

Chamblin Bookmine
Chamblin's Uptown
Jacksonville, FL.

Laughing and Loving with Autism

All marketing and publishing rights guaranteed to and reserved by:

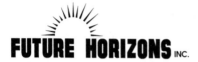

FUTURE HORIZONS INC.

721 W. Abram Street
Arlington, Texas 76013
800-489-0727
817-277-0727
817-277-2270 (fax)
E-mail: info@futurehorizons-autism.com
www.FutureHorizons-autism.com

Typesetting: Christopher Gepp—Austin, Texas

Cartoons and layout: Sue Lynn Cotton—Bedford, Texas

ISBN 1-885477-04-X

Dedication

There are many who deserve recognition for this book but clearly the parents, families and friends of children and adults with autism are the real authors and heroes in the challenge of autism.

Then, there is Alex, my autistic son. My time with him in his 16 years has taught me volumes about myself, my limits and the joy of unqualified love. His unique perspective of the world and his efforts to be better have earned my respect.

Next, but no less important, to my daughter Jennifer, who is often normal but never boring. Then there is my business partner, Polly, who has accepted the time given to this book and the Autism Society with grace and patience.

Finally, to my sister Dorothy, who would have loved this book. I like to think that somewhere, in a better place, she is enjoying her nephew's stories and smiling.

About the Author(s)

The author(s) is an amalgamation of family members, friends, and teachers of children and adults from all over America and the world.

Many of the stories are about my son, Alex, whose charm and often surprising perspective on the world formed the genesis for this book. I would relate "Alex stories" to my friends who encouraged committing them to print. Then as I spoke to others involved with autism, I realized that Alex was a microcosm of those with the challenge of autism. Countless others had stories equally funny and/or touching.

I then advertised in the Autism Society of America periodical, the *Advocate*, for contributions and received hundreds. It was "fun" work as I spent countless hours laughing, smiling and occasionally "tearing" at stories. My only regret was that they couldn't all be used.

Often, authors claim that their books are labors of love. That has never been as true as it is with this offering. The contributors show their greatest strength in facing autism: humor.

Introduction

To those of you not familiar with autism, let me explain what it is, and isn't, in very basic terms. It is not life threatening, rarely dangerous to others in any way and can't be "given" to anyone.

Autism is a developmental and communication disorder that acts as a block to "normal" interaction. It's as if a wall drops down around the autistic that interferes with the ability to communicate, feel or understand in "normal" ways. Nuances or subtleties are often lost on a child with autism because it requires too much in-depth understanding.

Where we understand a story or activity because of its "meaning", they listen to the words and literal interpretation of them. This "negative" is the basis for a lot of the humor—they see things exactly as they offered. In doing so, they often illustrate our own too-serious view of the same words or act. It's also worth adding that the word autism covers everything from those who are non-verbal and self-injurious to a few that graduate from college but still have serious problems applying skills because of the "communication wall."

There have been many books written on autism by knowledgeable professionals who have explored causes, "cures" and treatments of autism. Many of them had the first name of "Doctor" and have written with great depth and use of medical terms attempting to define and treat this mysterious disorder. Others have written from the perspective of the autistic or a family member. They have all, and usually with great skill, written in very serious terms about an admittedly serious subject.

However, if you want a book that labors on the pain of autism you're holding the wrong book. This writing emphasizes the unique views that persons with autism have of us, our values, our words and the things we feel are so serious. In fact, very often the humor is found in how they illuminate our "properties" and structured attitudes. A person with autism simply sees the obvious and relates to that image without being "hampered" by rules of our society. They see a world consumed by "saying the right thing." This gives them the freedom to see everything literally, and to speak honestly when we normal people would hold our tongues.

No one questions that all parents to autistic children would prefer to have the handicap removed. Yet no parent, sibling, teacher or friend does not balance that desire by drawing comfort from the love and laughter that gives us strength. We share the following anecdotes and stories so you can feel the positives of this challenge, and the joys that our "handicapped" loves bring to our lives.

This is a book intended to be a source of smiles, laughter, sharing and maybe a few warm tears—relax and enjoy.

Laughing

Many of the stories are about my son Alex and I've put those in this typeface. This way, you can trace common trends in his vision of our world. All other stories are followed by the name of the person who so graciously offered the anecdote. For the most part, the stories are in their own words. My occasional commentary is in this typeface as well.

As mentioned earlier, no one questions the challenge of autism. However it is equally true that these children and adults can suddenly offer a ray of humor that brightens our day. These offerings are representative of the humor "from left field" that often brings us back to the reality of their perspective.

Laughing

"A Lesson In 'Proper?' Identifications"

My son Jason Steele is 4 years old and is mildly autistic. His language is very literal and some of his "observations" are amusing. He does not intend to be making jokes, he simply labels things as he sees them—often more accurately than his parents do.

For instance, he saw a row of highchairs at a restaurant, but he didn't know the word "highchair" So, he pointed to them and accurately called them "baby sitters."

One day he openly resented being called a cowboy because as he said, "I ride a horse not a cow, so I'm a 'horseboy'."

Last fall, Jason properly changed the name for the greenbelt behind our house and said it was now the "yellowbelt."

Jason can't label all the fruits, but he knows strawberry and raspberry. So a lemon is a "yellowberry," a lime is a "greenberry," and a miniature marshmallow is a "whiteberry."

Jean Jasinski
Colorado

"Dr. Doolittle, I Presume...."

My non-verbal son, Peter, and I went to the New Mexico State Fair. We came to an enclosure where they were offering camel rides. He indicated that he would like to do this, so he climbed aboard an elaborately adorned camel. Peter, an adult, has very little speech but makes a happy growling sound when he is enjoying himself. I watched him and the attendant circle the yard. At the far end they stopped for a little while, and I wondered what was up.

When they came back to me, the attendant said in amazement, "Do you see that camel across the way?" referring to a dust-covered camel standing up against the fence. She continued, "We have been trying all morning to get that camel to stand up. When your son came by, making that sound, the lazy camel got right up because that is the kind of noise camels make."

I decided that a good job for my son would be awakening and communicating with camels, helped by a job coach, of course.

Elizabeth Hirsch
New Mexico

"But If It Could, What Would It Say?"

After several years of hard work with my son Michael, he was finally doing fairly well fitting into the community. For his eleventh birthday I took him with me to the bakery to let him order his cake himself, with the cartoon characters he preferred. He did really

4

well answering questions, like what flavor, frosting color and filling he wanted. His face pressed up against the glass as he surveyed the options. You could tell he was losing patience, though, when the lady asked him what wanted the cake to say.

He glanced up at her and said, "Are you crazy? Cakes can't talk! Just give me that one!"

Leah Devulder
California

♦♦♦

Children with autism will rarely lie, or, if they do, they do it very poorly and are delightfully confused when the "shallow" untruth us not accepted. Here are several stories that speak to this.

When my son, Chris Purdue, was 16 years old, he attended a moderately handicapped program based in a large high school. This particular class was on the first floor of the school, and, since it dealt with abstract concepts about money, he was rather bored. Also, he always loves to be up high, wherever he goes. Consequently, one day instead of going into the class where he was supposed to be, he decided to attend another class on the second floor to see if it was more interesting!

When the teacher came into the classroom and saw Chris sitting in a chair, she asked him, "Well, who are you?" Chris, who has good language and appears normal, sat up proudly and said,

"My name is Craig Alexander." (Chris knew another boy named Craig — where he got Alexander, who knows?)

Looking a little surprised, the teacher then said, "Craig, I don't think you belong here — you must be in the wrong room." Chris replied with assurance, "No, I'm in the right room — I've been here before." The teacher said, "No, I don't think so — if you'd been here before, I'd have seen you." Chris then said, "No, you're wrong. I've been here before. You've just not seen me because sometimes I'm invisible."

The teacher was very confused, the class loved it, and Chris never could understand how the teacher knew he didn't belong in that class.

Bev Purdue
Indiana

Buddy loves music and goes around the house singing Christmas songs in October. Sometimes, when alone in his room he can get real loud, singing while pounding on his furniture and toys. When you have to tell him to stop, he says it wasn't him. He always seems surprised when I assure him I know he's the guilty party!

Peggy Hitchcock
Ohio

One day, to my shock, Alex came to dinner with no socks on:

"Alex, you're barefoot. You can't come to dinner like that. At least put on some socks."

"But, Dad, if I drop food, I'll get my socks dirty!"

Sometimes Alex's "logic" is difficult to counter.

✦✦✦

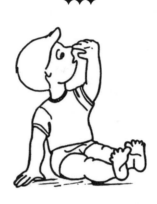

Alex was "stimming," rocking back and forth waving his arms, as I was telling him the story of Pinocchio and how his nose grew when he lied:

"Alex you can stop stimming."

"Dad, I'm not doing anything."

"You were stimming."

"Was not."

Then, after a thought raced across his face and with a look of fear, Alex slowly raised his finger up to touch his nose.

✦✦✦

Children with autism prefer things to be constant. Change is generally not fun. That point is brought out clearly here.

In our family, a favored weekend activity for my husband, Jim, and our seven-year-old son, Tim, who has autism, is to go for hikes on the nature trails in the city parks. This is followed by a trip to McDonald's. Naturally, this trip involves a very specific park exit to a very specific McDonald's. One Saturday, Jim attempted to vary the routine by taking a different exit. Tim became upset and protested against this course of action Jim tried to calm Tim, telling him that different was not wrong.

Tim replied. "But Dad, to me, it is."

Nora Rege
Oregon

My son Jason asked his bald father when he was going to grow more hair on his head. His dad tried to explain that he had hair once, but it fell out and he wouldn't be able to grow any more hair.

For a brief second, Jason looked confused. Then he looked down at his father's arms and hands and, confident that he had figured out the loss, said, "It's okay, Dad, it fell on your arms."

Jean Jasinski
Colorado

Doing his best unintended imitation of Jack Nicholson from Five Easy Pieces, one day Alex set a waitress back a bit by saying, "I'll have a ham and cheese sandwich but no ham and no cheese!"

My son, Sam, is a unique individual first. He has a wonderful sense of humor, a happy spirit and a willing smile. He likes to "play jokes." His latest is to stick his finger in his ear and say, "Oh no! Ear eat finger!"

He also likes to do "hi-five," which is a great improvement over the routine bite that he used to use as a greeting.

Anne Russell
Texas

"Just Don't Go to the Library with Her....."

Anne Marie plans to take care of me in my old age and has announced this to the staff at her group home, the Jay Nolan Center. She was recently very irritated with her roommate and hit her on the head with a book. After being reprimanded for this, she was quiet for a moment and then remarked to a staff member, "Maybe I shouldn't take care of my Mom when she's old, after all."

Margaret Pothoff
California

When my now 13 year old son was three, he fell in love with legos and assembled and disassembled them whenever he had an opportunity. One day as we waited at the doctor's office, he was engaging in his favorite exercise. Suddenly, he stopped cold as a worried expression crossed his face. He slowly turned toward me and reached up and tugged at my ears, nose and throat. With a sigh (I hope of relief), he said, "Not work. No take apart Mommy."

This was given at a workshop at an Indianapolis conference. Author Unknown

✦✦✦

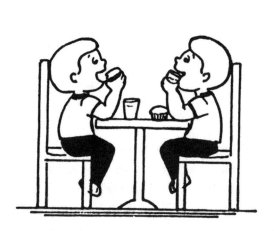

"Double Your Pleasure...."

My twin boys, Mathieu and Albert, age 6, are both autistic. However, they seem to show a willingness to share and help each other even though they do not with other children.

Each has his own food preferences. Mathieu likes potatoes, and Albert likes carrots. At dinner it is not unusual for the twins to finish eating their preferred food, get up simultaneously, walk around the table, sit at the other's place, and continue eating their preferred food from the other's plate.

When I mention it is time for juice and muffins as a late snack, Albert will get two juice cups and place them on the table and go to the fridge to get the juice jug and put it on the table. Mathieu will get a plate from the cupboard and put the box of muffins on the table. Mathieu will eat his muffin, and Albert will drink his juice. They then swap positions. Mathieu will continue eating Albert's muffin, and Albert will continue to drink Mathieu's juice. There is no problem of "what's mine" with them. Everything seems to be common property to be shared with his brother.

Harry Laudie
Quebec, Canada

◆◆◆

Our political structure is not always completely understood by those with autism. The following two stories will never make it to a political science class, but they do offer an interesting view.

My 29-year-old son Chris has always had compulsions regarding government, dates, and presidents. (He knows all the presidents names and dates of terms in office.) He insists on voting each year and spends days and months considering his choices.

I think the list he made for himself for the 1998 election is self-explanatory, characteristically autistic, and amusing especially his reluctance to vote for a woman.

1998 Primary

1. I will only vote for President.

2. I will vote for a man if possible, even if nasty.

3. Among the men I will vote for a nice candidate.

4. I favor Gary Heart. *(sic)*

5. I will see if there is anyone that I like better than Gary Heart.

6. I will put the candidates in order.

7. If possible I will vote for someone better than Gary Heart.

8. If possible I will vote for someone of my dreams.

Carol H. Benjamin
Virginia

Dear Senator Domenici,

I'm asking you to clean up New Mexico.
I'm a 5th grader in Mrs. Kline's Class.
My name is Allison Daggett.
I think the Wipp project should be abolished and that you should work to clean the air.
I also think that more solar power plants should be put in New

Mexico.

You should try to get people to stop throwing trash around and start recycling.

To make a long story short, I want you to clean up.

Seriously,
Allison

P.S. You can call my mom at 291-9738.

Diana Daggett
New Mexico

My husband and I were thrilled when our autistic son, Andy, learned to count. Once gaining this skill, Andy would repeat it time and again in any way he could. A little boring after the 400th time but we were still pleased with his new ability. Then we received our monthly phone bill with $38.00 in calls to South Bend, Indiana. We didn't know anyone in South Bend but the number was somehow strangely familiar.

Then we realized that to dial South Bend from our Northwest Indiana home, you need to dial a "one" first. That made the phone number 1-234-5678

Andy had spent $38 practicing his new skill every time my back was turned.

I tried to call the number to apologize, but it had been disconnected. I wonder why?

Jayne Kranc
Indiana

"Here we Go Again"

Uh-oh. There's a pregnant lady, and Buzz is headed toward her. Then comes his question and her answer that we have grown to expect:

"Are you cranky?"

"What??"

Actually, Buzz is asking a logical question. My autistic son Buzz was 3-1/2 years old when his brother Stephen was born. The days before labor pains began were hot and sticky, and I was in a really bad mood fussing at poor little Buzzy and the world in general all day long.

I hadn't been that grouchy before or since then (honest!), but Buzz will not let me forget how I acted on that day sixteen years ago. And whenever he sees any of our expectant friends, he'll ask her if she's cranky.

Taking a poll, I guess.

Sandy Grabman
Oklahoma

◆◆◆

Those that are higher functioning often have interesting interactions with businesses, particularly when they write letters. The first is a letter to a company with which many of you may have had dealings. The first letter's P.S. is priceless. The letter in the second story must have rattled some folks after the "imaginative" correspondence went out.

Dear Columbia House,

Buying these 12 tapes plus the other 8 means I must pay $89.70

I understand that I can buy these 8 tapes within 3 years.

If you make me pay any more than the stated amount, so God help me, I'll sue.

Sincerely,

Allison Daggett

P.S. After this, I'm canceling my membership.

P.S.S. Even though I'm only 12, you'd better take me seriously.

My brother, David Sudbury, is high functioning but still definitely offers some very "autistic-like" behaviors. Recently, he got a job, (he's had many) with one company working in their print and reproduction room. Things were going reasonably well until the president noticed some very unusual mail coming in to their address.

The mail was not to their company, Smith and Martin, but to Smith and Sudbury, attention David Sudbury, Vice President!

You guessed it, David had changed the company name to a more "appropriate" title and had appointed himself to an executive position in the process. He was happily directing things to be accomplished that he felt were best.

The President was furious and stormed into David's area waving a piece of the "creative" stationary in his hand. He found David in the middle of a copying project. The boss exploded as he stammered, "Give me one reason why I should not fire you right now!"

David, very calmly, answered the question exactly as asked, "Because I'm working on this job at the moment."

As you may imagine, he no longer works for Smith and Martin or, for that matter, Smith and Sudbury either.

Donna Lane
Florida

◆◆◆

"Instant Family??"

Our kids with autism understand more than we give them credit for and sometimes they find ingenious ways to reveal this.

When we moved to California from another state, I took our son David (then age 22) to the Regional Center office for the required physical exam and psychological testing. These appointments were scheduled half an hour apart. David was with me during the history taking part of his physical. The M.D. asked me if we had another children. I replied, "No." He then asked why we'd never had any more children. I said I'd rather not discuss that in front of my son, and he dropped the issue.

Then we moved on to meet the psychologist in another office. After giving David the required I.Q. tests, etc and having a conversation with David, he had me come into his office privately to answer more questions about my son's early years. He asked how David had adjusted to the move from another state. I said, "So far, so good." Then he asked, "And how are your other children adjusting?" I explained that David was our only child and inquired as to what made him think I had other children. I practically fell off the chair when I realized what my son had done. David had told him he had 10 brothers and 2 sisters!!

So, I ask you to remember this true story when you think of all the times you see that blank stare or you think they're in another world. Sometimes our kids with autism can show us just how sensitive to our feelings they can be.

Lorrain Groom
California

✦✦✦

Our son one day showed us his own unique application of the word autism. I was driving, with Buzz in the back seat, past a series of businesses. The bank had, as do many companies, an electric sign that scrolls words that offer a thought or an ad. Suddenly, he shouted. "Look Dad, that sign is autistic!" I turned to see that it was saying over and over "Have a....", "Have a....", "Have a...".

Ray Grabman
Oklahoma

✦✦✦

My son Ryan is now twelve. About three years ago he became fascinated with ages. (I think he knows the ages of most people in our small town.)

One day he asked, "How many years ago was Daddy 16?" I replied "Many years ago."

"How many?"

"Many."

"Well, was that before Jesus was born?"

Kathi Kopyn
California

We were dressing for Halloween and I was concerned that my son understood that this was an act, a game and not real. I don't think I got through to him. I dressed as a witch and he was to be a tiger. He was patient with the process but his attitude toward me seemed to change as I put on the last touches of my make-up. I knew he wasn't clear on non-transformation when he suddenly brightened with an idea, ran to the corner where we kept the broom, handed it to me and said, "Okay, now fly!"

Offered in an ASA conference workshop
Sorry, author unknown

I am a speech therapist at Sherwood Center in Kansas City. A couple of incidents always make me chuckle when I think of them.

One class of our older autistic students was copying a poem entitled "February Twilight" from the board. When asked, "What does 'twilight' mean?" one of the older boys showed the impact of Rod Serling as he quickly replied, "It's a zone."

Another time, one classroom was drawing faces "Draw some eyes," I said. So, one of my boys drew

Julie Thomas
Missouri

◆◆◆

Sometimes Christmas presents can have different meanings to different people...

It has always been the tradition in our family to give each child one "big present" (meaning it cost about $50) and several lesser ones for Christmas. The kids choose what that present is to be, since I'm not about to spend that much money on something I'm not sure they would like.

One October, my son Buzz told me he wanted a los Angeles telephone book for Christmas. That seemed reasonable to me, since he loves to collect phonebooks from other cities.

When I called the phone company to order the L.A. book, though, I was informed that it consisted of two separate volumes and cost far more than the allotted $50. Well, I thought, I'll go ahead and order it, giving him one volume on Christmas and the other on his birthday a month later.

It put a dent in my budget, to be sure, but I knew it would be worth it when he would joyously read through his much-desired new L.A. phonebook.

He did indeed seem pleased with his present. So I was very surprised when he took them to the local Chamber of Commerce office the day after his birthday and returned with an old beat-up L.A. phone book. I couldn't understand what had happened and was feeling a little hurt.

He patiently explained to his rather dense mom: He needed the new phone books to give the Chamber of Commerce so they would let him have their old one. The old one is much better, he said, because it has an illustration of the old Holiday Inn sign in its Yellow Pages.

Buzz never liked Holiday Inn's new sign.

Sandy Grabman
Oklahoma

◆◆◆

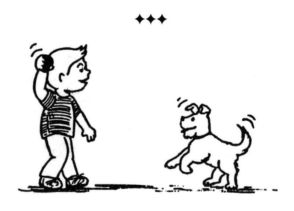

I've always been a pet lover and I was a little sad that Alex took very little interest in any of the family pets. However, one day I thought that there was a sudden awakening of normal interest.

I was tossing the rubber ball from the living room out into the hallway (this is something bachelors can do with impunity) so our very energetic dog, Spencer, could retrieve it, a game he loves. After about 5 or 6 tosses, I noticed a real interest in Alex's face as he followed every movement. To my further surprise, he asked if he could do it. I was delighted and Alex proceeded to throw with some vigor, whizzing the ball past Spencer out into the hallway.

However, after three or four throws, I saw that he was bothered and giving a sigh of disgust after each throw. Naturally, I asked Alex what was wrong. He was throwing the ball, with Spencer happily bringing it back so he could chase it again. What could be wrong?

"What's the problem, Alex?"

"Dad, I'm missing.... because Spencer keeps moving his head!"

There was poor Spencer, thinking it was a great game, never realizing that, in Alex's mind, he was a target.

No one can possibly calculate the positive impact of the movie Rain Man. Although not typical of very many autistics, Dustin Hoffman's part offered the general public an introduction to a world most have never known. The following article from the Hollywood Reporter and subsequent humorous and touching stories *sent to us by a parent of the Oklahoma and Bernie Rimland, one of the founders of the Autism Society of America, gives you some idea of the movie's impact.*

In a letter to the film's star, Dustin Hoffman, 12-year-old autistic Brent Aden wrote, after seeing the film, "...People care about autism now... I feel good now. People say autism is OK. I'm free now. This is good Rain Man."

According to Brent's uncle, Dan Wilkins, before *Rain Man*, Brent would respond only to the name Wally Cleaver. He called his uncle Kip Cleaver, his father Beaver, his mother June and his brother Eddie Haskell. Wilkins once lost Brent in a grocery store and had to have him paged as Wally Cleaver.

"Brent has always been ashamed of being autistic, but *Rain Man* legitimized his handicap," said Wilkins. "When he saw his hero Dustin Hoffman playing an autistic man, it clicked in him that it was OK to be autistic."

(*Hollywood Reporter*, March 28, 1989, Andrea King "*Rain Man* brings brighter days to autistic, families")

My wife and I decided to take our 18-year-old autistic son Buzz to see *Rain Man*. We weren't sure how he'd respond or how much he'd understand. However, our respect for his understanding grew as he watched the movie intently muttering under his breath, "I do that , I do that, I don't do that anymore...What's funny about that?"

Ray Grabman
Oklahoma

A mother told me that her eight-year-old son was really quite embarrassed, and somewhat depressed, about his autistic sibling. He was so ashamed that he didn't invite friends to his house after school and in general kept pretty much to himself.

After seeing *Rain Man*, he became quite elated and went to the teacher the following morning to ask to be able to share his autistic sibling with his classmates. After telling them that he was the brother of an autistic youngster, and about *Rain Man*, he capped his story proudly explaining that in the film, "Tom Cruise played my part!"

Bernard Rimland, Ph.D.
California

◆◆◆

"What's in a Name?"

Often, people who are not associated with autism "hear" the word with very interesting interpretations. Consider these.

Prior to moving to a new school district, I spoke to the principal over the phone explaining John's autism. Later, as we completed the routine paperwork, she asked, "Just what is an acoustic child?"

We considered taking in a foreign exchange student. I was concerned how our potential guest would react to John, so I emphasized his challenge in the information package. I thought that would probably end the issue, but to my surprise, I received a response several weeks later that the young girl in question was delighted because she, too, was "artistic."

Beth Sposato
Nebraska

Music

All children with autism, almost without exception, love music. The following stories highlight that love.

Music

Alex loves singing and was in his sixth grade chorus. It came time for Christmas recital. The group practiced for weeks and Alex, who has an incredible memory for songs, knew every song perfectly. To add to the excitement, the recital was to be held in the town square of Chapel Hill, N.C. in front of a large crowd. Finally, the big night came and Alex assumed his place in the group.

The recital began and the chorus proceeded to sing its repertory. However, amazingly, Alex didn't open his mouth to sing but simply stood there with a big smile on his face! His mother Starla was obviously a little taken aback and anxious to find out the problem. After the recital she worked her way through the crowd to Alex's side. Before she could say a word, Alex said, "Wasn't it good, Mom? Did you like it?"

Her confusion only increased. Starla said, "But Alex, you didn't sing a word."

Alex looked up with that look of surprise and said, "I might not have looked like I was singing, but I was...I was singing inside." After a moment of reflection, she smiled, gave him a big hug, and took her "silent singer" home.

When Alex was in the second grade, he loved music of all kinds but mostly rock, with his favorite singer being George Michael.

As it was the beginning of the Christmas season, his teacher *polled the class on their favorite song. The first said, "Rudolph the Red Nosed Reindeer," the second said, "Away in the Manger," the third brightly said, "Good King Wenselslaus." Then she asked, "Alex, can you tell us your favorite song?" He looked up at her, with his bright blue eyes, blond hair, and completely innocent face and said, "I Want Your Sex" (George Michael's big 1988 hit). The teacher could barely contain herself and the aide had to leave the room she was laughing so hard.*

Alex was singing in class one day and when his teacher asked him if he liked to sing he said, "Yes, I do. My voice is good. This voice was meant to sing!"

"Do You Need Whitney If You Have Rusty?"

I'm a mother of a three-and-a-half-year-old diagnosed PDD/autistic. He doesn't speak eighty percent of the time. But, Rusty does have some non-meaningful speech. If Rusty is in a particularly good mood, he will sit with a smile on his face and do "hand-flapping" and just say "diga diga diga"...over and over.

One day we went out for an afternoon drive. As usual, we were listening to music. Rusty was sitting in his booster seat, the warm Hawaii breeze blowing in his face; he began to "flap" and "diga, diga, diga." About that time an advertisement came over the radio for the Whitney Houston movie *The Bodyguard*.

They played a part of her new song where she sings, "I will always love you." Well, the "you" part is high-pitched and stretched out. Rusty continued "flapping" but suddenly changed his "song" to "diga, diga, diga...you!!"

The "you" was a perfectly pitched Whitney Houston imitation and exactly the right length! My husband and I rolled! This lovely memory stayed with our family.

Carla Clancy
Hawaii

◆◆◆

My husband, one of the Spinners, and I have a son with autism. Purvis is virtually non-verbal except, amazingly, when he hears the Spinner songs, he will join in singing every word with clear language and perfectly in beat.

Claudreen Jackson
Michigan

◆◆◆

"Memory Is a Wonderful Singing Skill..."

Jean-Paul did not have real language till he was almost 5, but he loved music and was able to sing many songs. Not surprisingly, his first purposeful speech was echoed lines from songs. One day, we visited a farm, and Jean-Paul wanted to climb up on a tractor. He turned to me, reached out a hand and sang, "With a little help from my friends" (from the Beatles). After I helped him up on the tractor, he sang, "Mr. Spaceman, won't you please take me along for a ride?" (from the Birds). We consider this some of his first meaningful speech.

When Jean-Paul was a freshman in college, it was the thrill of his music-obsessed life when the boys on his dorm floor organized a rock band. He was the lead singer and they named the band Jean-Paul and the 6-Pack. Their theme song was "Jean-Paul Be Good," an adapted version of "Johnny Be Good." Jean-Paul didn't like me coming to hear him sing, but when I heard they were doing a concert, it was just too exciting to resist. I sneaked into the performance to see the band.

I was hidden among the crowd of students in the college union, and I could overhear the comments of the young people. They laughed at Jean-Paul. His voice wasn't bad, but J-P moved in his own jerky, awkward way. There were comments about his "Pineapple Shirt," which he apparently wore constantly. I began to wonder why the "way cool" band members would want Jean-Paul in their band, so I asked the band leader. He sheepishly told me that they needed Jean-Paul because he was the only one that knew all the words to all the songs.

Julie Donnelly
Missouri

◆◆◆

This story is about why my autistic son, Michael, calls all angels "Gloria".

It all began in Cedar Rapids, a Christmastime long ago. There was a house with a fascinating Christmas display. It outdid all others in the area and was Michael's "most favorite."

There were angels, most of them holding choir books, but all with halos and open-mouthed, singing. I softly joined their chorus of "Glo-oooo-oh-oooo-oh-oooo-o-ria! In Excelsis Deo."

Michael asked, "What is it that they sing?" I said, "Gloria." We both gazed at the magnificent holy display.

And somewhere between listening to the lyrics and looking at the display, Michael decided that all angels, forever more, were to be called "Gloria."

M. Pat Mitchell
Iowa

✦✦✦

Sexual / "Improper" Language

Our autistic loved ones are often bemused and unimpressed by our preoccupation with sex and "improper" language.

Sexual / "Improper" Language

My husband and I were making love when we suddenly realized that our 13-year-old autistic son had quietly opened the door and was watching with a seemingly confused look on his face. We were both shocked and very concerned as to Dan's reaction. Hurriedly putting on my robe, I went to see Dan, who had gone into the kitchen, and was making a sandwich. The revealing conversation went like this:

"Dan, are you okay?"

"Yes" (as he continued on his sandwich creation).

"I want to tell you that Mother and Dad love each other and what you saw was one way we show it."

"Okay."

I didn't think his "okay" matched my anxiety so I continued.

"In fact, Dan, that's how we made you...by our love."

"Okay" (no expression).

Still feeling like I wasn't getting through and not knowing how to end it, I asked a leading question.

"Do you think you'd like to do that one day? Show love like that?"

Shaking his head and with a sigh...

"Nope...looks too much like hard work!"

Name Withheld at Mother's Request

"Way to Ruin a Guy's Thanksgiving..."

Anne Marie's father and I were divorced and several years later I remarried. As my new husband was going to be in the town where Anne Marie was going to school, I asked him to drive her home for Thanksgiving holiday. I thought this would give them a chance to become better acquainted.

As they began the trip, Anne Marie turned to him and calmly said, "Bill, I think you should know that Mother does not like sex." He said he certainly wouldn't want to upset her mother and, although he tried to appear calm, he soon found he was lost and had driven 10 miles out of his way.

Margaret Pothoff
California

♦♦♦

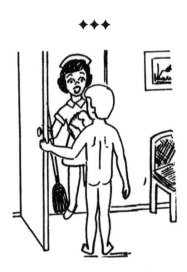

At about the age of 9 or 10, Alex was very immodest about keeping his clothes on. He just couldn't figure out why there was

all the fuss about garments if you felt good without them. One day we were at a suite-motel and were all dressing—except Alex—who was stark naked. The maid came to the door—Alex opened it and just stood there, looking at her blankly. She stared at our son, who was big for his age in every way. Finally, Alex said, in his curiously naive manner, "Do you want something?"

For some reason, she never came to clean our suite for the rest of our stay.

"We Think He Understands!"

I was watching a classic movie, the remake of *I Was a Teenage Werewolf*, with my autistic son. One of the characters suddenly spoke of scaring someone so bad that "they lost control of their bodily functions." Apprehensively, I asked him if he had any idea what that meant.

Without missing a beat or taking his eyes from the screen, he said, "Rusty zipper - yellow socks."

Mary Ann Coppola
New York

One time Alex, while traveling with his mother, maybe more accurately than he will ever know, referred to the Hawthorne Hotel as the "Hormone Hotel."

"A Lesson on French Toast"

When Robert was learning opposites and contrasts, I prompted him to say, "This is boy, not girl," "This is hot not cold," etc. He picked up on this quite well and we do it so much like a game that I sometimes talk autistic-ese.

One morning, I was fixing breakfast for Robert. I automatically started labeling, "This is regular toast, not french toast."

Some mornings later, Robert interrupted me from a snooze with a kiss on my cheek. He rubbed his nose and mouth on my cheek much longer than usual so I mumbled, "Just regular kiss, Robert." He mumbled back as he continued to kiss me, "Just regular kiss, not french kiss." I woke up real fast! For a minute, I was stunned. Who in God's name could have taught him about "french kiss"? My mind was reeling! Then, after an agonizing moment, I felt great relief as I remembered the lesson on french toast. Whew!!

Norma Page
Ahiog California

◆◆◆

I think one of the funniest things my six-year-old autistic son, J.J., has done was on a trip to the mountains.

We had checked into a motel and decided to go for a swim. After getting out of the pool and back to the room, I undressed J.J. to change him into dry clothes. No sooner did I turn my head than he made a mad dash for the door, ran down the hall naked. Seeing a door of another room slightly open, he swung open the door and immediately started jumping up and down on the persons' bed, laughing, stark naked.

The lady in the room was getting ready for dinner and came out of the bathroom in her slip to join her husband, who had been down the hall getting ice. In absolute shock, they were watching this naked stranger-child, who hadn't been there seconds before, frolicking on their bed. The look on their faces is something I won't ever forget. I never laughed so hard.

Autism sure can have its funny moments!

Debbie Bedard
New Hampshire

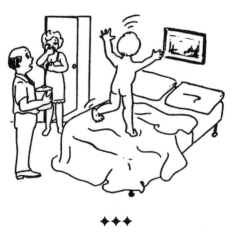

✦✦✦

My teenaged son not only "appears" to be normal, but immodestly I say (but with much input from others) is also a very good looking young man.

However, he very definitely acts autistic. This contrast led to a very interesting interaction. We went grocery shopping, proceeding to the checkout counter. The young lady ringing up our purchases was very obviously impressed with this tall, strapping young man and kept glancing his way as she rang up our bill. Since the glances didn't get a reaction, she looked at him and with a cute smile and eyes flirting, said - "How are you today?"

He snapped back from wherever he was, looked right at her and said enthusiastically, "Wednesday, I'm going to take a bath!"

She looked stunned as her mouth dropped open. He was satisfied with his response and I exited stage left as fast as possible but with a smile. I revisit that smile every time I think of her startled look.

Dottie Jurgens
Texas

◆◆◆

"Some Questions You Shouldn't Ask..."

In 1965, my daughter brought home her new husband to visit us for the first time. We were sitting in the living room getting acquainted when there was suddenly a loud pop in the next room. I, knowing what had happened, tried to ignore the noise and draw no attention to Peter. However, my son-in-law still looked concerned and asked what had happened. I tried again to defer but he was persistant. So, I reluctantly explained that Peter had learned the day before that if he climbed up on the end of the sofa, he could pee on the electric light bulb of the table lamp with astounding results and a wonderful explosion.

Our newest family member looked for all the world like he wished he hadn't asked the question.

Elizabeth Hirsch
New Mexico

"Safe Game"

My daughter, Anne Marie Bonnefil, told me one day that she never intended to marry or have a boyfriend. She firmly stated, "I guess you can just say 'Anne Marie's my name, and chastity's my game'."

Margaret Pothoff
California

"Where Do Kids Hear These Things...?"

My husband, my daughter with autism and I recently visited another branch of our family. This was a somewhat stressful visit for two reasons. First, it was at the home of the very proper matriarch of our family - our great aunt.   Second, they had offered that there really wasn't anything wrong with Beth that a little more "strict understanding" wouldn't work out.

Beth's appearance that day did nothing to allay that thought. She was dressed neatly and quietly assumed her place in the living room where we all sat around the aunt. All the proper conversation went on until Beth put her hand in the air and in perfect diction said, "Where is the goddamned bathroom?"

(The first thought that ran through my defensive mind was that everyone there knew my husband never talked like that, leaving a narrow choice as to where she heard that language.)

I quickly interceded with "Well, Beth - the gosh-darned bathroom is right down the gosh-darned hall, dear." They all ignored her outburst and I never again heard that Beth was absolutely normal.

Susan Moreno
Illinois

◆◆◆

"Girls...!!!???"

While our thirty-two-year-old son, Mitch, was on a home visit, I asked him, "Is there anything else I can do to help you?" Like most parents, I should tell you I've left no stone unturned to give Mitch all we can, so I was surprised by his answer, "Take better care of me."

I felt a little guilty and confused so I asked, "Son, what would you like me to do?"

You could have knocked me over with a feather as Mitch, looking very serious, said, "Get me girls to go to bed with."

I was literally almost speechless. I wasn't at all sure that this activity was in the mothers' handbook of responsibilities but was reasonably sure there was a name for it. I did the best I could with the situation by saying, "Maybe someday in the future." Thankfully, he accepted that answer.

Phyllis-Terri Gold, Ph.D.
New York

♦♦♦

Along with having a daughter with autism, I also teach students who have autism. One of them, Jeff, is very unpredictable and a real "free thinker." Recently, while walking down the hall, with a look of concern, but to no one in particular, Jeff blurted out, "I sure hope my penis is okay!"

Sandy Kownacki
Missouri

♦♦♦

"The Mystery of the Blue Light Special"

For several weeks, we had an unusual occurrence in that the pilot light in our gas clothes dryer was always going out. I was constantly finding it inoperative. It was a real puzzle.

Finally, we found that John, at just the right height, was putting the pilot light out in a very "unique" way. Our first clue was that John wasn't asking to go to the bathroom quite as much as usual.

Beth Sposato
Nebraska

Church

In our society, there are few areas where propriety is more strictly observed than in church or religion. Therefore, it is natural that it is the perfect place to have humor hit its mark.

Church

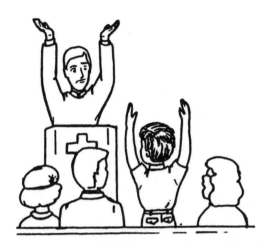

"Then why did he give the signal?"

When our son Chris was about 6, he developed an interest in televised football games. He would watch games standing in front of the TV and seemed to be very interested in all of the running, jumping, and falling. The slow motion replays would especially hold his attention. He'd flap his arms like autistic kids do, rock back and forth on his feet, and utter remarks like "Gee Whiz!", "Oh God!", "How could he drop that?" and "Fall Down!" At times he almost sounded like a Steeler fan.

Quite frequently after a play Chris would shout, "Touchdown!", imitating my victory chant whenever the Steelers scored. Most of the time, of course, a touchdown had not been made and I would say, "No Chris. That's no touchdown." He'd give me a perplexed look, and I never got the impression that he understood the difference between a touchdown or a first down or even a commercial. That is, not until one Sunday morning in church.

We got the bright idea that Chris might be more interested in religion if we sat in the front pew. At least we wouldn't have to worry about him stealing purses and wigs from the ladies sitting in front of us. It actually worked for a few weeks. Chris seemed to enjoy all the goings-on at the altar. He was especially interested in the organist and choir.

Chris had been watching the Mass very attentively. His eyes followed the priest as he walked toward our side of the church and stopped in front of us, raising both arms over his head to give us a blessing. Seeing this "signal," Chris jumped up and, in his loudest voice and clearest diction, shouted, "TOUCHDOWN!" The priest, with his arms still upraised, gave a startled look our way. I looked down at Chris reproachfully. He looked up at me and then "corrected" the situation as he shouted out, "That's no touchdown!"

Benoit Beaudoin
Pennsylvania

♦♦♦

"Love...ly Hymn"

One Saturday afternoon Robbie and I went shopping at our favorite store. The store's mascots are four Love Birds.

Robbie enjoys watching all animals and birds. This particular afternoon two of the Love Birds (Fred and Wilma) were grooming each other and Robbie got a big thrill out of this scene. Especially when I pretended to be the voices of Fred and Wilma singing, "I'll scratch your head, you'll scratch my chin, I'll scratch your back and you'll scratch my neck" (to the tune of "I'll Take the High Road, You'll Take the Low Road").

Well, it stayed with Robbie, for the next day was Sunday and right in the middle of church, as everyone else looked on with confusion, Robbie stood up and started singing "I'll scratch your head and you'll scratch my chin." My friends smiled gently and asked me on what page they could find this "interesting" hymn.

Valerie I. Rosica
Connecticut

◆◆◆

When our son, Mitch, had become a young man, he moved into his present group home. They habitually said Grace each night; each client was asked to thank God for the food before eating. One evening it became Mitch's turn. When he didn't say anything, one of the staff prompted, "Mitch, who do we thank for our food tonight?" Mitch answered, "I thank Bill."

Everyone was a little confused until they remembered that "Bill" was the cook. Great logic.

Phyllis-Terri Gold, Ph.D.
New York

◆◆◆

"'Refreshing' Visit to Church"

My 10-year-old son, Brian, enjoys going to church at least partially because of his love of music. So I take him to our Catholic service whenever possible. Normally, I take him in the side door after the service starts, quietly finding seats in the back.

However, one Sunday we walked in with everyone else because we were going with out-of-town guests.

Everything seemed to be going well as we proceeded into the narthex greeting other parishioners.

Everyone in front of us were quiet and respectful as they made the sign of the cross with the holy water. All was fine until suddenly Brian spotted the water. He loves swimming and taking baths takes a strong second.

Before I could reach him, Brian's eyes lit up and he plunged his face in the holy water and began blowing bubbles vigorously! Other than his sounds you could have heard a pin drop as everyone in the narthex froze. Then, just as quickly as he went in, his head came up evidencing a huge grin. He looked at me, said, "Good," and proceeded to take a seat in the last row.

Somehow, I didn't think God or the Catholic Church would mind.

Mira Blaine
Alberta, Canada

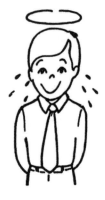

Ruth Sullivan is one of the founders of the Autism Society of America. She and her son Joe have been on "Oprah" and other talk shows. Joe was one of the models Dustin Hoffman used in preparing for his role in Rain Man. This story involves one of her trips to church with Joe.

We attended a confirmation service. At the end, the priest, in his red regalia and holy sceptre, left the altar and went slowly down the aisle to pleasantly but solemnly greet the parishioners as they left. As we were in the front of the church, we were among the last to leave but there was still a crowd around the priest as we got to the door. Without warning, Joe, with a smile, reached through the crowd to touch the priest and said in a loud voice, "French toast." Our otherwise verbal clergy wasn't sure how to answer that unusual greeting. I, on the other hand, aware that French toast was one of Joe's favorite things, knew that in his own way he was trying to say that he enjoyed the service.

Ruth Sullivan
West Virginia

◆◆◆

Our son's name is Mitchell Alan Goldberg. When he was very little, I used to pray aloud by his bedside each night. He gave me no indication that he was even hearing what I was saying, which always began, "Dear God, please help Mitch in all ways that you can and help us, too," etc, etc. This continued for about two years until one evening, when I sat down at the edge of his bed as usual,

Mitch startled me by telling me emphatically, "No Dear God tonight!" and promptly turned over to go to sleep.

Phyllis-Terri Gold, Ph.D.
New York

Facilitated
Communication

A new treatment that is intended to break down the walls of autism is Facilitated Communication. Although controversial in its applications, it has many advocates. Basically, it offers the non- or slightly verbal person an opportunity to communicate by typing on a keyboard with an aide assisting them. The following stories are about autistics communicating through Facilitated Communication.

Facilitated Communication

My son David communicates very well and often bluntly through facilitated communication. Recently he was working with his facilitator and a visitor who was assessing his skills. After several hours, she had completed her work but wasn't sure how to end the conversation. One question followed another as she sought an appropriate close, without success. Finally, she said, "David, is there anything else I should ask you?"

He quickly typed out, "No, just open your mouth and say goodbye."

Connie Deming
New York

◆◆◆

"Maybe He Was Just Being Polite..."

My brother, Phillip Rivkin, is autistic. Although he communicates somewhat through sounds and body language, he is non-verbal. He responds to people and understands a limited amount of cognitive information, so we thought. Until the recent discovery of Facilitated Communication to which he has responded in flying colors, my family and I did not have a clue to his inner life. He never read a book to our knowledge, yet his spelling and sentence structures are nearly perfect. His comprehension is amazingly clear and precise. His sensitivity and awareness to people and the world around him is that of a mature adult.

He loves to eat, particularly to go out to a restaurant and always (or so I thought) enjoys my choices of food style. In one of his typing sessions, I told him that we were going to go have lunch at a Chinese restaurant I had taken him to a multitude of times, more than any other place.

He stunned me with his typed reply: "I don't like Chinese food!" After all these years of assuming he adored Chinese food, I was shocked to learn something new about him. Naturally, I am glad he finally told me...even if it was thirty years later!!!

Lena Rivkin
California

My son, Jordan, was talking through F.C. to one of the group home leaders. She said she was going to give a speech on autism to a local group. Jordan asked her to tell him what she was going to say. She proceeded to give the outline of the speech, expecting a positive reply.

After she finished, he looked up, somewhat disdainfully, and typed onto the screen, "Maybe you'd better let me go instead."

Howard Weinroth
Toronto, Ontario

Home

Even in the sanctity and security of our homes, we are subject to the surprises that our special family members can offer. These anecdotes are fairly typical of how even everyday events can turn into fun experiences.

Home

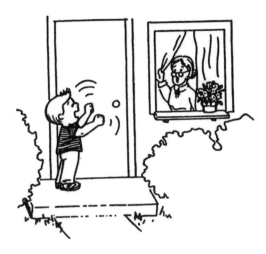

"'Murder' At Bondi - A Story of Nicholas Power"

The Sydney, Australia beachside suburb of Bondi is usually quiet on Sunday mornings during October. The swimming season had not yet quite begun and in the early morning not even busloads of tourists had arrived.

This was the scene recently when the peace was broken by a phone call to Bondi Police Station. A caller, new to the neighbourhood, frantically told the desk clerk that he feared a violent fight, or even worse, a murder was taking place in a house in Anglesea Street about a mile from the beach. A patrol car was dispatched and immediately sped to the scene. As the police arrived, the screams and banging could be heard shattering the calm of the street. With their experience of the "melting pot" at

Bondi, the police felt they could cope with whatever was happening inside the house and so lost no time gaining entry.

On this occasion, though, their experience came to zero. Upon entering the house, they expected to be met by a deranged murderer, axe or dagger in hand. They were instead confronted by Nicholas, a young autistic boy of 11 years, whose daily routine is to let out ear-piercing, blood-curdling screams, while banging on doors with both his fists, all the time maintaining a happy, angelic expression. He was only letting off steam.

The new neighbour was not aware that situated in Anglesea Street was a respite care house for disabled children.

Nicholas was not arrested, fingerprinted or had his mug shots taken—in fact, Nicholas was quite a celebrity. He is also known locally as "The Granny Terroriser" due to the fact that on the few occasions he has escaped from Anglesea Street, he is always found hooting and howling in a block of pensioner flats just up the road. The senior residents know him now and are besotted by his angelic looks even though initially, nobody was game to open their door.

The new neighbour is used to Nicholas' antics now—along with all his other noisy friends that attend Anglesea Street Houses—and no doubt wait with breath held for the next escapade.

Paul & Coralie Power Bondi
Junction, Australia

◆◆◆

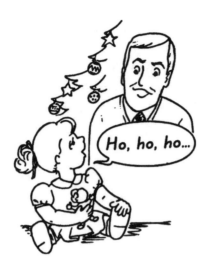

"A Christmas Gift"

When our beautiful little girl, Suzie, who has autism, was about five years old, her great-uncle came to visit us at Christmas. Not a terribly sensitive man, he jutted his thumb at Suzie and said gruffly, "Does she understand anything about Christmas?"

Suzie, heavily into self-stimulation, jolted back to our world. Sitting ramrod straight, she looked him directly in the eye and said defiantly, "Ho, ho, ho."

Suzie and her great-uncle have been the best of friends ever since.

Dennis and Diane
Focht Nebraska

Once Mitch, who lives in a group home, was visiting for the weekend. He got up in the middle of the night, apparently hungry and prepared himself his then favorite, and very messy snack, bread covered with ketchup. My husband, hearing Mitch in the kitchen, went in and, speaking somewhat sternly on seeing the ketchup mess, asked Mitch, "What are you doing!?" meaning, "You should not be making this mess!"

Mitch looked at my husband as if to say, "Are you stupid? What I am doing is obvious," but patiently he answered verbally, "I am eating bread and ketchup."

Phyllis-Terri Cold, Ph.D.
New York

◆◆◆

"Be Careful What You Ask For..."

About two years ago, my husband was struggling to listen to our son express himself on some subject. My son was having a hard time finding the right word, so my husband said, "Spit it out son!"

Seemed like a strange request to Shawn, but he did; stopped talking, spit, and then continued on trying to find the right word.

Sandra Phillips
Virginia

◆◆◆

"Put That Mouse Back in his Home!"

Before Christmas, we put up a wall "Countdown to Christmas" calendar in our son's room (when he was four). The idea is to move the Christmas mouse into the next numbered pouch each day, starting with 25 until you reach 1 day before Christmas. Each family member got their turn. However, when we had our son move it, he kept putting the mouse back to the 25, where he first saw it.

Robert & Susan
Cromwell Kansas

Alex, like most kids I suppose, continually left his clothes on his bedroom floor. Being a well-trained parent, I sailed into him with my best shot, a line I had heard from my parents and one that the reader has also probably heard. This was the interchange:

Dad - "Alex, this is the last time I'm going to tell you to pick up your clothes."

Alex - (With a sign of relief) "That's good, Dad, because I hate when you tell me that!"

"Maybe Also a Few Good Books and Valium?"

In order to keep my son out of rooms he was obsessed with, we had our doorknobs turned around backwards so we could lock the door easily. This worked until one day my daughter and I were both in the bathroom, bathing. I heard an ominous click and realized my son had just mastered a new skill.

Now we were frantically locked inside, hearing my son screetching through the house. Our imaginations ran wild as to what was happening on the other side of that door. We were finally freed after two very long hours to a kitchen that was deplorable. A gallon of spilled orange juice, an updumped box of cereal and many other contents of our refrigerator were strewn all over the floor. It was either laugh or cry, but, when I saw my son's happy and unharmed face, I started to laugh.

However, the next time we headed for a relaxing bath, we were accompanied by a telephone and bathrobes.

Carolyn Scheggia
Pennsylvania

♦♦♦

Not too long ago we were all in the car ready to go somewhere, except that my husband was still inside. After blowing the horn several times, I asked our autistic son Shawn to stick his head in the door and tell Dad to come on.

I looked up in a few minutes to find Shawn with his head pressed into the screen door, and he was calling his Dad, just like I'd asked him to do!

Sandra Phillips
Virginia

♦♦♦

As with my reasonably normal daughter, I always said "I love you" to Alex when tucking him in at night. After a while, he responded in rote fashion, "I love you too."

Being "clever," I said, "But I love you more," to which Alex quickly responded, "Then I love you less."

✦✦✦

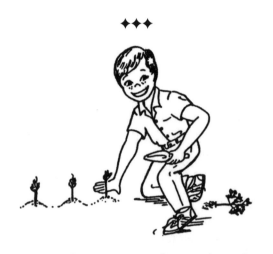

In 1972, Peter was living in a residence where they maintained a greenhouse. One morning he was assigned to bed young tomato plants. He was very careful how he set each plant the proper depth in each row. His supervisor left him for several minutes, and when he returned he found Peter, with a big grin on his face, carefully planting the seedlings in a neat row upside down, with the roots waving in the air.

Elizabeth S. Hirsch
New Mexico

✦✦✦

"Nite, Nite..."

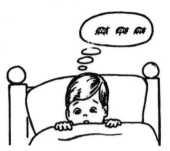

This story is about our son Mitchell, a high functioning autistic.

Growing up, there are a lot of "sayings" that parents tell their children. When you have your own children, you pass on the old traditions. Of course, if you have an autistic child you don't always think of the reaction before you speak. That was the case in this story.

Every night, my husband Johnny would put our son to bed. They would talk about Mitchell's day, then Johnny would say goodnight. One evening he added an old rhyme, but new to Mitchell: "Nite, nite; sleep tight; don't let the bed bugs bite."

Mitchell jerked up in bed and started frantically searching the bed for bugs. To any other child, the words would have meant little, but at that time, Mitchell was terrified of bugs. It took a while, but we finally managed to convince him that there weren't really any bugs in his bed.

Mitchell is now eight years old. He is still afraid of some bugs, but has learned to manage his fear and has changed a lot since the incident of two years ago. Now, the rhyme is a regular ritual at bed time. But I tickle him instead of looking for bugs.

However, one night I forgot. As I turned down the light,

I heard his voice behind me....."Nite, nite; sleep tight; don't let the bed bugs bite."

Jill Gentry
Kentucky

Alex's stepdad was encouraging him to bed with, "Last one in bed is a rotten egg," to which Alex responded, "Okay, what's the first one?"

✦✦✦

"I'll Make It Go Away..."

One of the most touching things that Jessica ever did was to try to wipe the frown lines from my forehead. Whenever I frowned (probably too often), she would take her little hand and try to smooth my forehead. It may not be classic therapy for frowns but it always worked.

Jennifer Brown
Ohio

✦✦✦

"Haven't We All Felt This Way?"

I stayed with my nephew, who has autism, while his mother and dad went away on a trip. I had the responsibility of waking him up in the morning, one he didn't appreciate. I shook him gently but firmly and said, "Time to wake up," to which he groggily replied, while trying to bury his head in the pillow, "Not wake up. Wake down, wake down."

Marjorie Speakman
California

✦✦✦

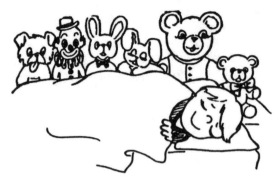

When our son was young, Joseph would go to bed without any problem and sleep through the night. We would tuck him in bed with one or two of his many stuffed animals, and say a prayer with him and then leave. Often, when we checked on him in the morning, all of his stuffed animals and dolls (about 20) would be in bed with him, all lined up precisely along the headboard!

Robert & Susan Cromwell
Kansas

◆◆◆

"The Boy Who Fell from Grace with His Mommy, and Took His Dad with Him"

What I am about to describe to you is not a pretty picture; a naked 15 year old boy sitting on the commode with his right foot stuck firmly to the floor. What, you might ask, would bring a young man to this abased circumstance?

Our son, Tom, is autistic, and among many other things that we have developed in order to manage his life and times, we allow him to buy bubble gum while we check out at the grocery store, depending on his behavior. Over the years, he has been the model of deportment, so buying his usual two-bit jawbreaker is practically a given.

Home we went, and we began our ordered routines: we, unpacking; he, preparing for his bath. At fifteen, we have gotten him to a point where he practically prepares himself for the bath/shower, a great improvement over even a year ago. This night, however, something was amiss.

No shower was running. My wife, Megan, just knew something was wrong.

I grunted my acknowledgement as she moved off to the silent bathroom. The silence was broken by a frightening sentence, "Honey, you have to see this to believe it."

What a sight. There was my naked son, with his foot stuck to the floor, pieces of gum in his hair, on the wall, his fingers, ear lobe, etc. He usually disposes of his huge wad of gum easily, but this night he must have dropped it, stepped on it and tried to dislodge himself from the shag carpet.

So, there we were, two fully grown butlers, trying to clean up the mess around him, Tom was still seated with me at his feet trying to wipe gum off his foot with kleenex while MY foot kept sticking to pieces of gum on the floor.   Meanwhile, Megan, surely trying to be helpful, was behind me, alternately berating Tom for his behavior and me for my ineptness at correcting the situation.

Ah well. Another of life's lessons. Did you know Crisco gets gum off vinyl floors? I didn't.

You see, Megan wound up having to use Crisco in the shower stall, as Tom repaired to the tub at his Mommy's prompting (I'm being polite here) before the gum was off his foot or his hands.

Needless to say, Tom is "grounded" for two weeks; that is to say, no bubble gum for two weeks. And, my feet stopped sticking to the floor this afternoon.

Harry Richards
Pennsylvania

✦✦✦

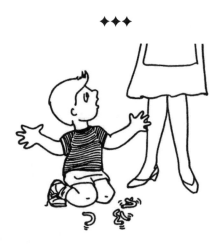

When my non-verbal son Peter was five years old, we were living on a farm in Maryland. One day he came to me from outside, grabbed my hand, and indicated that he wanted me to do something for him. I followed him and found that he was engaged in his favorite pastime: lining up or printing the alphabet. However, this time, he was trying to do this by making the alphabet out of live angle worms. Sadly for Peter, the worms weren't being too cooperative. A and B were crawling away while he was making C Needless to say, this was one time that I couldn't do what he wanted.

Elizabeth Hirsch
New Mexico

✦✦✦

Shortly after we moved to a new house in a different state, my mother came to visit us. Our autistic son, three-and-one-half years old, got out of his recliner chair and walked over to his grandmother shortly after she entered the house. "How nice!" we thought. He even grabbed her hand! Terrific—a sign of affection! However, then he escorted her right back to the front door and indicated she could leave. She did not belong here!

We reassured Mother she was wanted. However, shortly after that, he again took her hand, but this time he walked her to his bedroom and left her in there, closing the door. (He has done this with us, too.)

Robert & Susan Cromwell
Kansas

◆◆◆

"Who's Sorry Now?"

When John was in high school, there was an incident one day in which he mangled a teacher's eye glasses.   It was, of course, very inappropriate and unacceptable behavior and could not be ignored.   It seemed right that she should be compensated for the new frames that were required.   It didn't seem entirely right that John should get off with no obligation while his parents paid for his destructive act.   He should pay. Yet his earning power was practically non-existent—until a snowfall conveniently arrived soon after the incident.

"John," I announced, "you are going to shovel snow because you must pay for those glasses you broke."   I showed him the sidewalks that were to be shoveled and he started in on the task. I was rather surprised at how cooperative and compliant he was. I had expected more resistance to this demand. Inside the house, while he shoveled away outside, I felt rather pleased. Not only that I had done the right thing, but it was easier than I had expected it to be. Later, I went out to look at the job he had done.

The sidewalks were acceptably cleared.

The snow had been piled into a small mountain inside the garage.

Beth Sposato
Nebraska

"Definitely Not a Fat Cat"

My little friend Jeff's mother was very concerned about the amount of food the cat was eating but without gaining any weight. Worried, she took him to the vet who informed her that, in fact, the cat was starving.

It wasn't until she found it necessary to replace the vacuum cleaner bag that the mystery was solved. Turns out that Jeff loved the sound of the cat food being sucked up into the vacuum. Hence, the constantly clean plate cat bowl.

One can only wonder what the poor cat must have thought of the sight of his food disappearing into a tube.

Sandy Kownacki
Missouri

Out into the "Real" World

It is not only necessary but very important that we parents of children with autism venture out into the public. Trips, whether to the grocery store or to another state, become much more "exciting" than with our normal children. We're never quite sure how our special kids are going to perceive an event or how the general public is going to react to our kids. The following stories are about some of those adventures.

Out into the "Real" World

"Sarah's Shopping Spree"

I went shopping with my 14-year-old autistic child, and, as happens with all parents, I "momentarily" lost sight of Sarah. I quickly scanned the parking lot and surrounding area, then returned to the store wondering if she might be looking for me. There was still no sign of her. Finally, in desperation, I hurried to the checkout line.

At first, I was very relieved to see her but my comfort quickly dissipated as I realized that she was calmly putting her "purchases" on the conveyor. The cashier was just as calmly ringing up her order. In only a few minutes, Sarah had completely filled her shopping cart with a variety of her favorite items. One problem! Sarah had no money! I announced to the cashier rather sheepishly that she was my daughter but those were not my groceries. I apologized profusely and hastily exited the premises with my errant progeny but without her "wish list" groceries.

Fisher family
Michigan

◆◆◆

Many children with autism "perseverate" or focus on a subject almost to the exclusion of other interests. For too long of a time Alex focused on bathrooms. That's all he wanted to talk about. One day while driving in the country, I had about all I could take of toilets, sinks, and urinals and snapped at my son, "That's it. No more talk of bathrooms for at least an hour. We're going to talk about something else,....like that airplane up there."

For one brief second, Alex looked taken aback and then peering up at the plane, he brightened up and said, "Now, Dad, that airplane has wings, seats, and a neat bathroom." Then catching my scowl at the last item he'd mentioned: "I guess you made a mistake by talking about that plane when you knew it had a bathroom on it."

Very often, friends can be so absorbed in their own lives that the actions of our children can be interpreted by them as being "normal." This story illustrates that point.

Little league baseball is a torturous experience for me at best.

However, my normal baseball-playing son wants to see his adoring mother's face cheering him on every time he looks up. Then there is Darrell, our 10-year-old who is autistic. He finds sitting that length of time difficult and the constant eruption of noise even more so. About five games into the season, a friend of ours, Bob, sat down to watch the game.

Bob began to tell me how frustrated he was, having been an accountant for years and now, having to look for a job, was unable to find one in his field.

Darrell was playing with the strap of my purse and sucking his tongue.

Bob went on to say that, in his desperation, he took a job in the meat department of a local grocery store.

Darrell was now sliding up and down on the bench. I had a vice grip on him as I tried to be attentive.

Bob finished his story, "It is incredibly cold back there. The meat is heavier to carry than you would imagine and the floors are wet. Someone could slip and all for minimum wage!"

At that moment, a chuckling sound emerged from Darrell's throat, growing louder until he was laughing outright.

In horror at the inappropriateness of it all, I said, "Darrell!"

At which point, Bob took Darrell's hand and said, "That's all right, Son. I thought it was a big joke, too. That's why I quit."

I wasn't quite sure who needed my help.

Pamela McGee
Georgia

◆◆◆

"There Has to Be an Easier Way..."

Scott, my normally non-verbal son, and I were returning home from another unpleasant meeting regarding self-abuse and inappropriate behaviors. I had four lanes to cross over to get to the lane I needed. Suddenly, the traffic stopped dead and I ran into the back of a brand-new van. Scott's forehead hit the windshield. He immediately rubbed his head, looked at me, and said, "Oh."

I was so pleased with his talking, I forgot the accident for a moment and said, "So, this is what I have to do to get a word from you." He continued rubbing his forehead and laughed. I really want Scott to be verbal. I'm just not sure running into automobiles every day is the best way to make it happen.

Patricia Harman
Ohio

◆◆◆

"Take My Sister - Doc - Please"

Both of my autistic children were afraid of doctors. Any trip to the doctor was a dreaded experience. One Saturday morning Jessica had to go to the doctor to have stitches removed. Her brother Richard had to come along with us. I assured him that the doctor was not going to look at him, only Jessica. When the doctor walked into the room, Richard grabbed Jessica and shoved her at the doctor. He wasn't taking any chances that the doctor might be confused and treat the wrong child.

Jennifer Brown
Ohio

◆◆◆

When Scott was around twelve years old (and talking in three and four word sentences), one of his pleasures was to go to our local Lunch Rooms (Dru & Bill's), sit on the same stool and order the same thing (hamburger with potato chips and a Coke). Well, one day Scott put his order in and waited to be served, sitting

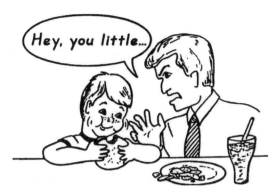

between two other patrons. I turned to talk to someone else and suddenly heard "HEY, YOU LITTLE WISE ASS!!!" The man commenced to grab Scott by the arm with the look of "I'll fix you" on his face.

I jumped up, placed myself between Scott and the irate man and demanded he tell me why he was accosting my son. The not-so-gentle (at the moment) man went on to say that Scott reached over, grabbed his hamburger, took a big bite, and put it back in the man's dish right under his gaping mouth.

I tried to explain Scott's handicap and offered what I'm sure was Scott's reasoning. "I ordered a hamburger. There's a hamburger. I'LL EAT IT!!!" So he did! By this time, the man was more composed and understanding. When Scott's hamburger came, I gave it to the gentleman. Scott just went on eating the man's hamburger, appearing oblivious to what was going on around him.

A happy ending, I might add. The man paid for our lunch!!!

Jean F. Butler
Maine

◆◆◆

Four years ago when my daughter, Julia, was four years old, we decided to take a Sunday drive to the picturesque town called Sedona. Julia was finally toilet-trained (after several attempts) so we didn't need to bring the diapers.

Everything went well on our outing until we decided that it was probably about time to have Julia visit the restrooms.

The restrooms we remembered from our previous trips to Sedona were no longer there.

A clerk in a gift shop directed us to the "outhouses" three blocks away.

When we arrived at the outhouse—a new experience for my daughter—I explained to Julia, "You go in here and go potty." She looked a little confused but proceeded to do as she heard me direct. I guess it was my fault for leaving out some information. Julia went inside, just stood there, and went on the floor, fully clothed. I forgot to be more explicit and say to undress and sit down.

Mary Turnquist
Arizona

◆◆◆

Our family was attending a local high school football game. Michael, our 12-year-old autistic son, seemed to be learning some of the basic concepts of football, as well as enjoying the game clock. All those numbers counting down on the clock, in that nice orderly fashion...it was heaven to him.

It was about a minute before half time and the score was tied.

The people in the immediate crowd around us were commenting on what a great game it was and trying to guess our team's strategy. We had the ball, but had a long way to go to score a touchdown with only 52 seconds left in the half.

My husband commented to a small group of people in front of himself, Michael, and me, "Well, we better get ready for the bomb." Everyone accepted that "grandstand coaching" idea, except Michael; the look on his face was one of near panic, as if he were ready to run out of the stadium.

"There's going to be a bomb, an explosion?" he said to me, seated on his other side.

I knew I had to talk fast in order to avoid chasing him on a dead run out of the stadium. I quickly explained to him that "the football is called a bomb when you throw it a long way for someone on your team to catch. There's not going to be an explosion, it's just a funny way to talk about football."

In a few seconds Michael was calm, but I did notice those peculiar looks he gave me three or four times in the next few minutes. I don't know if he really believed my explanation or does he ever?

Maureen Sharp
Iowa

"I'll Drink to That..."

At a large family picnic in a local city park, I suddenly discovered that my son Todd, who experiences autism, had disappeared. He had joined another group of people. A woman was pouring drinks and setting them along the side of a picnic table.   As fast as she poured, Todd was going behind her, picking up each cup and drinking the contents.   She stopped pouring with an alarmed look on her face.

Todd was waiting for more as I retrieved him, apologized and returned him to our family picnic.

Vahrlene Crosswhite
Missouri

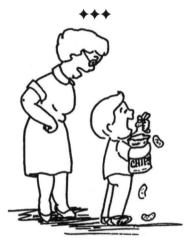

Our son Ryan is a seventeen-year-old severely handicapped/ low-functioning autistic individual who loves junk food. Consider this comical story from about ten years back.

Ryan's mom and grandma made a quick trip to the market one Saturday afternoon, taking him along for the ride. They parked the car directly in front of the store and briefly "ran in" to pick up a couple of items leaving Ryan to himself in the backseat. Certainly no big deal...right? After all, the store front was all glass creating a perfect view and the car was locked with Ryan not more than twenty feet away. It was only for a minute or two.

Well, it must have been a very intense motivating factor for Ryan when a lady pulled into the parking space along side with several bags of groceries visibly perched on the back seat. We think it was the sight of that sack of potato chips protruding out the top that prompted Ryan to learn how to unlock those car doors and rapidly plunge into the rear seat of that lady's car before she even had a chance to get out. He was "lightning" fast in ripping open that bag and proceeding to stuff those chips into his mouth with both hands full. When Mom and Grandma glanced out to witness, they claim that the expression on that lady's face could never be described short of capturing it on film.

But certainly this was no time for pictures. An explanation was going to be tough enough.

Brad Dietz
Michigan

◆◆◆

Sometimes the patience of a stranger can be very helpful in an otherwise potentially embarassing situation.

When our son Loudie was about seven or eight, I took him to McDonald's for lunch. It was always a challenge to balance a tray of food with my infant daughter and my flapping, non-verbal, autistic son. As I stood at the counter, waiting to order, I was surprised to see Loudie with a coke that he was enjoying and a much-surprised patron who never saw his coke disappear. Unfortunately, he was hungry as well as thirsty. At my next glance he was gone. He had planted himself in the lap of an elderly gentleman and was consuming his french fries with both hands. I ran over blabbering that my son had a communication problem and really didn't understand what he was doing. The elderly gentleman smiled as he responded, "Maam, I think he's communicating pretty well. He just looks like a hungry lad to me."

Carolyn Scheggia
Pennsylvania

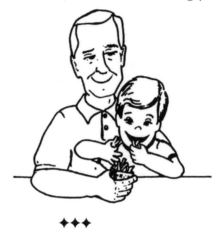

♦♦♦

Many young people with autism have impressive "splinter" skills, an ability to do something in an exceptional way that a normal person could never do. This story is about a rather unusual "skill."

Our son Mike is a good-looking young man. A casual observer would never know he had such a severe disability as autism. This is a blessing—and sometimes not such a blessing. As with most of these children, he always had something to perseverate on, and at the age of twelve he caught bees. Remarkably/ he could spot one yards away and would race to catch it in flightl He would hold it by its wings, observe it for while, and then release it to fly away. Mike never got stang and rarely hurt the bee.

One day our doorbell rang and it was the neighbor from down the street who had just moved in with his wife and mother-in-law. He said, "I don't know about that son of yours!" I responded, "I don't either, but what has he done now?" He fumed that Mike had been peeking in their windows and had really upset his mother-in-law. I looked toward his house and immediately understood. The hedge across the front of his house was in full bloom! I explained that Mike only wanted to catch the bees on the man's flowers and wasn't at all interested in what or who was in the house.

Our new neighbor walked away with a puzzled look on his face—probably thinking there were not just one, but two, strange people living here.

Monica Moran
Texas

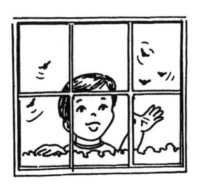

✦✦✦

"We All Need a Life!"

Attention mothers:

You know you've been around your autistic child too long when you go to a fast food restaurant and order a pink milkshake! When our son David was a pre-schooler, he had no difficulty learning his colors, but he could not pronounce words with several syllables. So when we were teaching him the difference between strawberry (his favorite), chocolate, and vanilla ice cream, he called them pink, brown, and white. So, David and I had our own milkshake code and we had it down pat.

One day on a McDonald's visit after I'd placed our takeout order, the cashier looked at me blankly and said, "And a pink milkshake?" before it dawned on this tired-out Mom what I'd said!

Mothers beware: you need to get out of the house more often (I know it's not easy) and converse with other adults occasionally.

Lorraine Groom
California

"Litter-ly"

In an attempt to teach my children how important it is to "Keep America Beautiful," I have been strict to enforce no littering to my autistic son Jeff who enjoyed throwing things out of the car window. One day, as we were driving to the mall, much to my surprise, Jeff excitedly said, "I just saw a sign that says that it's okay to litter." I assured him that couldn't be true. He replied, "Yeah, Mom, the sign said 'Fine for Littering.' It is okay to throw stuff!"

Ann Buckenstaff
Missouri

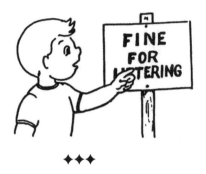

FINE
FOR
LITTERING

◆◆◆

"Fore?"

Our son, Joshua, is 5 years old with a smile that can light up your day and a loving disposition. He is also autistic and a "runner." This fall we spent a weekend in Orlando as we visited Disneyworld.

The first day we thought we would "relax" by the pool and let our kids enjoy a swim, one of Josh's favorite activities.

Relaxation ended, though, when I noticed that Josh had discovered an exit behind the pool area that led towards a small road and the golf course. We immediately rushed and attempted to catch up to him (in our bathing suits, I might add). Josh took off running with a clear determination of where he was going.

Once I realized he was into the golf course, I stopped (not wanting to interfere with the players and conscientious of my "attire"). My husband, John, of course, had no choice but to continue after him towards the 18th green where a group of four distinguished, elderly gentlemen were ready to putt. Joshua rushed through the group as if they weren't there, picked up the flag, and proceeded to run with it much like an Olympic runner carrying the torch.

As John grabbed Joshua, put the flag back, and apologized, I could do nothing else but laugh as I watched the look of confusion on the speechless gentlemen.

Terri Osman
Florida

✦✦✦

One day I took Alex, who at the age of four, was very echolalic (repeating back whatever he heard) with me to an IBM computer exhibition. As we went through the door to the hall, loaded with all kinds of IBM equipment, we were greeted by the perfect IBM prototype salesman. Well trained, perfectly groomed, ready for every event - except Alex. No IBM school prepared this guy for what he was about to encounter.

John IBM quickly sized us up and, as I'm sure he was trained, said hello to me and directed himself to Alex, bending down to his level. The conversation was priceless.

John - Hello, how are you?

Alex - Hello, how are you?

John - My name is John, what's yours?

Alex - My name is John, what's yours?

John - Isn't that neat. We both have the same name.

Alex - We both have the same name.

John - Well, John, I'm with IBM and I want to welcome you.

Alex - I want to welcome you.

A mask fell over John's face - what in God's name was going on? I was just standing there smiling with no intention of resolving a thing - this was fun! John took another tact.

John - Would you like a lollipop?

Alex - Would you like a lollipop?

John - Well, I have some. I was offering you.

Alex - I was offering you.

John - Well, I have some.

Alex - I have some.

John looked confused and knew the IBM manual had failed him.

John - Well, John, I'll see you around the show.

Alex - I'll see you around the show.

Numerous times, as I and my walking recorder strolled around the hall, John would go by and sing out, "How you doing, John?" only to hear his words come right back at him. John would smile, sure he was scoring points, and move on. The obvious never dawned on him.

"Good Choice?"

After working on my daughter Amy's teeth, the dentist told Amy to pick out something she want to take home (meaning any item from his prize box).   Amy promptly turned around, took the dentist by the hand and led him to the door.

I wasn't sure whether she planned to take him home to torture him or because she felt he was the best item there!

Sandy Kownacki
Missouri

School

Turning our children loose in an educational atmosphere offers untold opportunities for laughter. The structures required in a school are usually fine with our kids as long as they meet the guidelines of what our children, in their unique way, consider to be sensible. When they don't meet that test, look out! You'll all enjoy these but if you're a teacher or educational professional, you're really going to love the following.

School

I was helping Alex with his homework when we got to Math. The drill required learning math terms with the first being "hypothesis." Since Alex has a problem with things that are not concrete, I thought this was beyond him, but I tried anyway. "Alex, it's an idea that could happen." I explained it as basically as I could. He regarded me with a blank stare.

Later, to my chagrin, there was a recap exercise. The first question was, "Make up your own hypothesis." I turned to Alex without much hope. "Alex, you have to give me a hypothesis."

He replied, "Maybe I will."

Sometimes I wonder...

"Gotcha!"

Ryan's dad is a seventh grade regular education teacher in Sioux City, Iowa. Our son, Ryan, is in his class. This situation can be awkward for any parent/child, but with Ryan's willingness to say whatever pops into his mind, it can be "dangerous" to the parent. Mark had put on a few extra pounds over this past winter, and Ryan likes to tease his father about this.

One day Mark was talking to his class and stated, "Guess what I saw the other day for the first time in a long time?" Ryan replied, "Your feet?"

Mark and Barbara Renfro
Iowa

+++

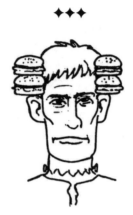

Alex had to write a story for English (very difficult for Alex) on any subject. Here is his offering on the subject he chose—one of literature's classic "monsters."

Once there was a monster named Frankenstein.

He lives on Franklin St.

He likes to scare people and make them run away.

Every Friday, he goes to McDonald's to eat 100 hamburgers.

Frank cooks his burgers with electricity and puts them on his ears.

+++

"Newton's Law"

Recently, my seven-year-old son, Tim, had his first playground accident at school, falling from some bleachers and acquiring a few scrapes. In attempting to find out how high he had been climbing, I asked him, "How far did you fall?"

Tim gave me that tolerant look he uses for silly questions and replied, "All the way, Mom."

Nora Rege
Oregon

Jessica had a great fascination with perfume from a very early age and an amazing ability to tell one from another. She always stopped by perfume counters and requested certain fragrances. A spray from a perfume bottle was a favorite reward.

When she was 5 years old she started attending a new school. She walked into the classroom, went up to the woman who would be her classroom aide, smelled her wrist and accurately announced "Estee Lauder." The aide was shocked and impressed by this charming but unusual skill.

Jennifer Brown
Ohio

When Alex completed elementary school, he told everyone he got to walk across the stage and meet the principal...who gave him his "gift" certificate!!

"Never Stand Between a Boy and His.....Calendar?"

One of my autistic students, Jay, is a stocky five-year-old who kicked and scratched his way through the first few weeks of kindergarten. However, happily for all of us, his behavior began to improve when he fell in love with the calendar. In fact, Jay's first words were "One, two, three" as he pointed to the calendar.

Jay spent his free time with the calendar. If he was having a problem with schedule changes or a difficult new task, the calendar would calm him down. The calendar was the center of Jay's school day.

We received a call one morning that Jay's bus was pulled off along the interstate and would be late. We thought it was engine trouble until Jay appeared at the door dwarfed by two large, uniformed security guards. They were holding Jay's chubby little arms firmly as if he were a serious criminal. One guard said, "This little boy rushed the bus driver, grabbed the steering wheel and scared that driver to death. Almost wrecked the bus."

The other guard added, "Doesn't like school, huh? Guess he was trying to turn that bus around and go home."

During our brief conversation I learned that the bus had taken a detour. I asked the guards to release Jay. They reluctantly let go and stood back. I wasn't surprised when he threw off his coat and ran for the calendar shouting, "One, two, three".

I try to educate people who come in contact with autism for the first time, and I did try to explain to the guards that it wasn't an aversion to school that had caused Jay's seemingly terrorist act, but a fear that the bus was going to take him away from school and his beloved calendar.

They shook their heads and listened politely as they backed towards the door. As they hurried down the hall, one of the guards looked over his shoulder and said, "Good luck, lady."

Tom Flowers
Teacher
Indiana

"Buddy"

This story is about my son Buddy who is thirteen years old. He is multi-disabled besides having autism. He is at a middle school now. One day at school, this kid was teasing him and even hitting him. So Buddy took his school bag and hit the kid with it. As life is not always fair, it was Buddy who got in-school suspension all day long in one room. He even had to eat his lunch in the room. He came home from school that day and said to me, "Mom, that in-school suspension is not fun at all. It's boring, and you can't leave the room. Why do we do it?"

Peggy Hitchcock
Ohio

Often, having a child with autism causes an otherwise normal parent to respond to a situation in abnormal ways. Peg says the story is about her son, I'm not so sure.

The story is about my son, Bobby, who is attending a four-year-old pre-primary classroom for kids with all kinds of disabilities. Every day the teacher sends home a note explaining his behavior that day. One day his teacher, Mrs. Lynne Munson, sent home a note that critically pointed out "Bobby was spitting on friends today."

I read the note, but unlike the average parent who may have been upset or angry, I was delighted. I started to hug Bobby and jump up and down yelling, "Bobby, you have friends. You have friends!"

Peg & Tim Jindra
Michigan

◆◆◆

The story involves my son, Scot, who is now nineteen (19) years old, and who is now and always has been very verbal, but exhibits many autistic-like behaviors.

At the time of the story, Scot was eight or nine years old and was attending a special-ed class for students with autism. One of Scot's friends in that class was a cute little Oriental boy whose name was Michael. Since Scot had a very definite fixation with school buses, this was his favorite topic of conversation, especially at the dinner table.

One evening, during such a conversation at the dinner table, his bus story centered around Michael. At one point in the story, Scot said, "Michael rides a handicapped bus." To encourage his continuing the conversation and, also, to see what his response would be, I said to him, "Is Michael handicapped?" He looked at me with a look of total disbelief, to think that I could ask such a question, and he replied emphatically, "NO, HE'S CHINESE!"

Betty Manning
Virginia

I was informed by Alex's special education teacher that Alex was to receive an award at the 7th grade awards ceremony. It was with a mixture of pride and apprehension that I took my seat. How would he act going up on the stage? What would this mean to him? My concern increased as I realized that his seat was all the way in the back of the auditorium, requiring a long trip down three aisles to get to the stage.

The proceedings moved on with all the 7th graders receiving awards in everything from academics and sports to service to the school. They all, being seventh graders, accepted their awards looking at their feet, the ceiling, their best friend, etc, saying very little or nothing and leaving the stage.

Finally, it was Alex's turn. The teacher began, "This next award is for a very special young man. When I was told I was going to have a student with autism, I didn't know what to expect. Alex has been a joy. He's very mannerly, sweet and tries his very best. This award is for Alex Gilpin for effort, manners and attitude."

I turned to see the biggest smile I've ever seen coming down the aisle. His loping walk was far quicker than usual and he negotiated the path to the stage perfectly. He shook the hand of the teacher and turned to leave. However, he stopped dead in his tracks. My heart stopped along with his stride. What was wrong? Then he turned and did something no other student had managed. In a voice loud enough to be heard in the back of the auditorium, he said, "Thank you. Thank you very much!"

There must be an air pollution problem in that auditorium because my eyes were very misty.

No, Alex, thank you. Thank you very much!

Poignant

When I began the book, I didn't visualize this section, but many stories arrived that were not humorous but were touching and warm. After all, wasn't this to be Laughing **and** Loving with Autism? *So, for your pleasure, here are offerings that give another perspective and a sensitive side to autism.*

These stories also unintentionally reveal as much about the courage and hope of the writer as they tell us about their subject...

Poignant

My normal grandson, Jeff, and I had just been to see *Aladdin*. As we drove home I asked him what three wishes he'd ask of the genie if he had the lamp. With no hesitation at all, he said, "First, I'd ask him to take away my brother Andrew's autism and then I'd ask him to take away my Grandmom's Alzheimer's."

He paused a while, so I asked, "And what about the third wish? Something for yourself?"

"No, I think that would be enough, Pop," he said.

This from the nine-year-old brother of an autistic four-year-old.

Bill Hale
Virginia

One time, after I had admonished Alex about something, he and I had this conversation that shows how an autistic child will zero in to try to understand emotion:

Alex- Do you like me?

Dad- You mean love...of course I love you.

Alex- No- I know you love me, but do you like me?

Alex, in a discussion with his mother, tried to explain (without realizing he was doing so) his challenge with autism. This was the conversation:

Alex- My brain doesn't work so good.

Mother- Now, or all the time?

Alex- All the time.

Mother- Mine doesn't either.

Alex- How doesn't yours?

Mother- Remembering names. Why doesn't yours?

Alex- I don't know—I just can't make it think sometimes.

Starla Clement
North Carolina

Another conversation with me, shows the literal and, in a sense, realistic, way Alex treats emotions. His mother and I, who are divorced, discussed Alex moving in with me. We were concerned how he would react to that idea, so I offered the idea innocently and was shocked by the response.

Dad- Alex, do you want to live with me?

Alex- Yes, I would...if my mother dies.

Dad- I, uh, well, um, uh—how would that make you feel? Would you miss your mother if she died?

Alex- Occasionally.

I decided to commit to paper my experience with Jean Paul, both pleasant and less pleasant. It was a sometimes difficult experience as I relived the entire process. After completing it, I had the history of Paul in a folder on my desk. He came in, found it and wanted to read it. I was very apprehensive about his reaction but took a deep breath and handed it to him.

After finishing, he gave little reaction, so I asked what he thought. "Sounds good, Mom."

Then realizing he may want to have a part in the story, I asked what he thought we should name it. He paused for only a second and said, "The Adventures of Jean Paul." It came to me almost instantly that it was a perfect name. My interactions with him were sometimes painful but they were always an adventure, one I'm glad is a significant part of my life.

Julie Donnelly
Missouri

"David: A Different Kind of Miracle"

A child's kiss, a hug, saying "I love you." As parents, we expect this from our children. We take simple things for granted. My son, David, has taught me not to take anything for granted. Not even little things. However, I've learned that miracles do happen.

David is 7 years old, tall for his age with thick brown hair, a dark complexion, and beautiful eyes. David is exceptionally cute and adorable.

David is autistic.

When he was younger, he did not like to be held or touched. He didn't talk. He would just sit alone in his room spinning the wheels on his toy dump truck. No one else existed to him. When he was two, I tried to force him to let me hold and rock him. He screamed and began hitting and kicking me. I was devastated. We took him from professional to professional to try to find out what was wrong with him. They would all say the same thing: "He's fine, he's just behind developmentally." One doctor even told me, "There's nothing wrong with him, you're just over-protective." Well, when he was three, we finally found out what was wrong. "You're son is autistic."

I have learned so much from my son. To take things one day at a time and never give up hope. David has so much determination. I've watched him struggle just to make eye contact. He would know what he wanted but had great difficulty saying it. One of the happiest moments of my life was when he stood in front of me, reached his arms up in the air, and said "hug."

David has shown me that there is more than one kind of miracle. He has so many miracles. He will always be autistic. He won't suddenly wake up one morning and be "normal." There are many things David can't do that other children his age can. That doesn't matter to me. In his own way, David can communicate, and love. He hugs and kisses, laughs and smiles, and he is happy. We have had a different kind of miracle.

My son David is now nine. He continues to make progress. The most important thing that I've learned from him is to never give up and not to overlook the other miracles in life that are a little different than the ones we may want. There are more important things in life.

Belinda Limbrock
Michigan

◆◆

This is written by a lovely girl who had a class project to write about someone who had made a significant impact in her life. Of all the people in her world, Tashana chose to write about her autistic step-brother. I'm sure you'll enjoy it. I've never met Tashana, but she appears to be an exceptionally sensitive and caring young lady.

It was November 9, 1988 when I received the news that my stepmother, Anita, was getting ready to have her baby. My aunt, my grandmother, my little brothers, and I waited at home for the news of the arrival. Then at 6:15 p.m. we got a call that my stepmother had a baby boy, and we decided to name him Alexander.

We were all so happy for her. The next day we went to the hospital to see the baby. I was the first one to hold him. He looked so adorable. We were all excited about having a little brother and looked forward to all the things you do with little brothers, play-talk and laugh. I got to know him really well, and he got to know me. I was like his second mother.

Then he started to have ear infections. We took him to the doctors and found out he had to have an operation on both ears. He was one year old. After the operation we noticed something different about him. So he was examined at the Kennedy Institute.

That's when they found out he had symptoms of autism, which is a disturbance in language and communication. He has picky eating habits, abnormal attachment to objects (like lining up cars), developmental delays in some areas (potty training, talking) and not in others (knows all commercials and all songs but doesn't seem to watch T.V.). Alexander goes to the Gateway School for hearing and speech-impaired children.

We now know that our expectation of having a "normal" brother is unrealistic. We have to take him to the bathroom, teach him how to play with toys, and how to put on his clothes and take them off. But I'm very helpful. I think he's starting to get it.

He's four years old now. He's learned new words in school and sign language for other words. He can't talk like any other four year old, but he's doing his best. And no matter what happens, we will always be there for him, and we will always love him.

Tashana Green (14 years old)
Maryland

◆◆◆

"This Is a Father...!"

I'm a single parent of an autistic boy, Travas.

He and I live in a rural area and have no access to other parents sharing parent/child stories about the trials and heartaches autism brings.

I can't rely on the public school system to benefit his needs nearly as much as I can give him at home.

Travas is low functioning; he's seventy-five percent toilet-trained, non-verbal, and has a short attention span. Handsigning is always implemented, yet no responses from him yet. We shower together daily and use hand-on-hand soaping and hair washing. We're presently working on how to use toilet paper.

Travas and I live in a large home in southern Utah on a three-acre ranch. We have horses, ATV's, sailboats, a lake ten minutes away, and much more. Sure, I enjoy these things but most of this is for Travas and his recreational needs. We have only each other under this roof. It can be lonely yet so fulfilling.

I'm not a wealthy man, but any and all extra money I receive goes into an account to better Travas and his world about him. Travas enjoys his trampoline, swing set, and, with the right luck, a swimming pool in 1995! He loves water.

P.S. Donny Osmond is a neighbor and enjoys singing to Travas almost as much as Travas loves hearing him! Mr. Osmond has a unique interest in Travas and often visits him. Travas has a unique interest in music.

Tony & Travas Tullius
Utah

◆◆◆

Challenging, different, loving, and small. All of these words describe Derek, who is so very unusual. Now, at the age of seven years and nine months old, he is beginning to communicate through facilitation (using an alphabet board to talk). He had come a long way. This type of communication may not seem very important to the majority of adults, but when you have a child who is very very special, you take what you can get and PRAY that someway, somehow, more progress will come along. Any miracle is welcome, even a small one.

He is a wonder to all. No one has any way of knowing what is really going through his mind. It is very obvious that he is intelligent. I can only assume what he may be thinking some times. The only thing I can say for sure is that Derek is unhappy because he has limited communication skills. Facilitation does not compensate for vocalizing, but shows the desire to talk.

Facilitation has eliminated a great deal of the pulling on Mom to demonstrate a need or want. Derek seems to be a happier person these days. He knows that he doesn't have to scream to get attention. He enjoys being around others and enjoys affection. He gives kisses to others, sometimes too freely, I think! He enjoys music and occasionally likes to be read to.

I consider myself and family blessed because things could be worse. I thank God for my children. In the Bible, The Lord says, "He would not have put anything on his people that they cannot bear." I truly believe this. I have been through a lot in my 31 years, and I'm still going through difficult times.

Bertha Gray
Virginia

"Sometimes a Walk in the Park is More Than a Walk in the Park..."

This true story is from a grandparent experience. My daughter is married and lives in Wortonga, Australia and has two children. James is "our" autistic child. I visit always my children every eighteen months, because I am very much interested. I do what I can for my children. I have been a member of ASA for years.

Several years ago I went to visit my daughter and her family. When I said I would like to go for a walk with James, my daughter replied that it was not such a good idea because he will not walk, he just takes off and runs. I went anyway. Boy, did I ask for it!

When I let go of his hand, off he went. I tried to catch him but could not because he was too fast. So I yelled, "Help me, fetch him," real loud. The other people looked at me, and all the kids went after him. They caught him and pinned him to the ground 'till I got there. I was out of breath, but I kneeled down and spoke to him: "James, we will walk, but you have to give me your hand and not let go or we go nowhere."

He gave me his hand, and we finished our walk out the park to the sidewalk to go home. When we hit the corner of the street they live on, he stopped and would not move an inch, went stiff like a board, and said, "Walk more, go more, no home." I said, "No, young man, I can't. We've got to go home for lunch."

He had a tantrum right there! So, I picked him up like a sack of flour and carried him home. He was screaming and kicking. His father came running to help. I said, "No, please. Let me take care of him. I am O.K." I didn't let go of him. I talked to him: "Oma

(Grandma) loves you, James. We are going home, dear one." As I arrived at the house, my blouse was all unbuttoned, my skirt ripped, my hair a mess, half-dead. But James and I had our first walk.

The next day I said, "You want to go for a walk again, James?" He came running to me, gave me his hand, and pulled me to the door. This was the beginning of our daily walks. After a few days of walking I let go of his hand, and he would walk in front of me. But I walked behind him, saying, "Wait for me, James. Don't run, wait, don't run." It worked. After four weeks, I left. He had learned to go for walks without running and even without my "coaching."

James is seven years old now and attends regular school and is a good student. He is a high-functioning autistic.

Recently, I saw him walking across the schoolyard to go home. I just stood there and cried, but with happiness for how he's come along since our first walk in the park.

Gertrude Schustek
California

♦♦♦

Many school districts actively practice inclusion, making every reasonable effort to expose handicapped, special children to normal children and vice-versa. However, other school districts do not. Nancy, eloquently and uniquely, speaks to the latter situation.

"Being You and Me"

One very snowy weekend at Deer Creek State Lodge changed three young boys' lives forever, not to mention all the adults who were privileged to be a part of the magical weekend.

They came together in the most natural of ways. "Eric, this is my son, Gabe. Gabe, this is Eric. How old are you? Do you like swimming? Gabe's ten, he swims like a fish. Would you like to join him after dinner?"

Eric seemed very timid about the water, especially the deep end. Every time Gabe got close, Eric felt compelled to inform me. I let him know that Gabe was a very good swimmer and actually preferred deeper water. Eric seemed surprised by that and took to keeping a closer eye on Gabe, not out of concern, but out of wonderment.

It was Saturday afternoon that I learned of Eric's near drowning incident just the year before. No wonder he was so cautious and so concerned about Gabe. As I watched the two parallel play, a pattern emerged. Gabe would swim up and allow a brief game of catch. Eric would follow Gabe to the deep end and swim from rope to ladder.

By dinner of the second day, the boys were best friends. Smiling faces were worn as they sought places together at the same table. Later, special toys were shared and a bond had been made that only young boys make.

Now for Brian. Because of the bad weather, Brian did not arrive until just before dinner Saturday night. All through the meal

Brian couldn't take his eyes off the two guys his age at the other table. Because of a busy schedule, hasty introductions were made. "Brian, this is Eric and this is Gabe. Gabe, Eric, this is Brian."

By breakfast on Sunday, Brian was visibly straining to spend time with the boys. He had mentioned to his mom what a cool dresser he thought Gabe was. Finally, the three met up and spent the snowy morning sharing toys and food and fun.

This story is only remarkable if you know that Gabe is a child with autism, and does very little communicating verbally. Eric is a kid who was afraid of the water and has epilepsy. Now Brian I'm not totally sure about. Basically, he has "eleven-year-oldism," which means he doesn't really care about autism and epilepsy. He thought Gabe was a cool dresser and Eric was a great guy.

When it was time to go, Eric was announcing how Gabe had taught him how to swim. Gabe was looking both Brian and Eric in the eye and smiling a lot, and Brian had made some new friends.

This story was so long in the telling because I can't get past the pain of why this thing called friendship can't happen every day for Gabe. After all, it really wasn't magic. It was three guys being allowed to be themselves, being cool, being eleven, being afraid. Given the God-given right to be "just friends," "why can't that happen every day?" In school, it happens for millions of children all the time. Unless, of course, you have a label and you have to go to special classrooms with other special kids, with special teachers who know special things. It's so special that this education never happens next to kids who don't really care about labels, or disabilities, but about just being a kid.

My pain is not just for my son, but is also for all the Erics and Brians who will never be allowed to know guys like Gabe, who won't be allowed to learn from his abilities, and be cool and be friends just because you want to and you can.

Nancy Ray
Ohio

◆◆◆

This letter to the editor was written by a high functioning young man with autism. I also received a copy of the actual letter. The handwriting may not win any penmanship awards but the sentiments in the letter win a "'hope" award.

Dear Editor,

I'm a 25-year-old young man who was born with autism, and I relate to the show "Life Goes On" because Corky, the main character of the show, played by Chris Burke, has Down's syndrome, like Burke himself. I personally think it's the best show on TV, but I want Howard Rosenberg to know that his lawyer brother is not alone in liking the show so much ("There's More to 'Life' Than Ratings," April 18).

If ABC does cancel that wonderful show, which I hope never happens, why doesn't the Family Channel on cable pick it up and make some new episodes? This will tell the many families of Down's syndrome children, as well as other disabled children, that there's a lot to learn from a Down's syndrome child, which is that he still has the ability to make it through life like the rest of us.

Jack and Marcia Cohen
California

"'Special' Special Kid"

You are my little special child,
My funny valentine,
An accident of Providence?
Or are you by design?

It matters not the answer,
For you are here with me.
That you're not like the other kids
Is mighty plain to see.

But you are a worthy person
Who has come a long, long way.
Helping you has helped me grow
To where I am today.

There's something I must tell you,
Though the words are nothing new.
They've been sung so many times,
I say them now to you.

Is your figure less than Greek?
Is your mouth a little weak?
When you open it to speak
Are you smart?

Though other folks may think you odd,
You're my favorite work of art.
 My funny little valentine,
You've slipped into my heart.

Claudreen Jackson
Michigan

◆◆◆

I realized how much laughter and joy Pete has brought us. His good humor and love of life lighten up our days. A quotation from G.K. Chesterton epitomizes his beliefs: "An adventure is an inconvenience rightly viewed." Rather than being annoyed when it rains, he views it as being an adventure. For him, falling down when skiing is almost as fun as not falling down. Since he has been home I have changed my attitude towards life entirely. Nothing "stresses" me anymore. I make a stupid mistake, I laugh. A broken egg on the floor is funnier than an intact egg. Every day with him brings laughter into our lives. Certainly throughout the years I have been frustrated, desperate, angry, hopeless, ready to give up, but after forty-nine years, the sum total of good times far outweighs all the bad times.

Elizabeth Hirsch
New Mexico

"FRIENDS"

When our son with autism was in his last year of public school there was an aide in his classroom whom Mike could really relate to. Mr. Craig was not much older than him, and Mike followed him around and imitated his every move—hands on hips, scratching his head, shooting the basketball—whatever Mr. Craig did, Mike did. Mr. Craig taught him the "High Five" handshake, and they greeted each other with it every day.

The school year ended, and Mike no longer saw his friend. A year passed, and the one day as Mike and I were leaving the shopping center, from across the parking lot came a loud "MIKE!" Mike looked up, saw Mr. Craig, and the two of them raced toward each other, and with big smiles gave the "High Five." What a thrill it was to see the joy on Mike's face at the surprise meeting with his friend!

Monica Moran
Texas

◆◆◆

"Ode To Scott"

Scott learned very quickly when he was just a little fellow to dress himself and brush his teeth.

"But he cannot tie his shoes."

Scott was slow in talking (seven or eight years old) but now (twenty-seven years old) has little difficulty in expressing himself.

"But he cannot tie his shoes."

He earns an "A" in hygiene, as he keeps himself well groomed.

"But he cannot tie his shoes."

Scott's athletic ability (especially bowling) is between the "norm" and the "above norm." He loves all sports and finds a way to play them alone.

"But he cannot tie his shoes."

He's kind, caring, and tries so hard to fathom his place in this new society.

"But he cannot tie his shoes."

Scott's a twenty-seven year old, whose growing ambition has now given in to working year round (Sheltered Workshop)—ONE GIANT STEP FOR THIS YOUNG MAN.

"But he cannot tie his shoes."

Scott operates our home computer, playing computer games, but mostly practices his typing lessons with 100% accuracy.

"But he cannot tie his shoes."

Last week, a friend of mine showed me a simple doubled knot way to tie a shoe. I, in turn, showed Scott this simple way, and he has been tying his shoes ever since.

"NOW HE CAN TIE HIS SHOES."

What's next Scott? It's up to you. You have climbed the Mountain of Despair with just a short distance to the "Summit of Success."

Go get 'em.

I am silently angered by some who seemingly choose not to recognize Scott's gains, from a serious "Autistic" cloud, to a slow, but definite climb in the right direction.

Jean Butler
Maine

"Opening the Cage Called Autism"

In his mind, there's a cage called autism.
Sir Apraxia's guarding the door.
Trapped inside, there's a wealth of knowledge

We never knew existed before.

A locksmith by the name of Crossley
Discovered a brand new key:
Facilitated Communication?
Sounds doubtful, but we'll see.

Oh my God!
The door is opening!
Apraxia's there, but he's stepping aside.
He's letting out all of the knowledge
That's been Kapped in this young man's mind.

The usual path's still impassable, though.
There's a road block on route to his mouth.
The detour signs lead elsewhere.
They say, "Go a little south."

The road from the mind to the arm
Is the new path knowledge will choose.
Go farther and there, find the fingers.
Yes, this is the route to be used.

Patricia A. Frank
New York

◆◆◆

*Some people with autism have high splinter skills but
still have problems interacting with our society. The
following contribution comes from such an individual.
Jerry has a math degree but has nor financially benefited
from that accomplishment. His words may give you
insight into a "savant" type with a different view of life
but a very poignant closing.*

◆◆◆

"Notes from a Missing Link: Welcome to My World"

I enjoy sharing my autistic history with groups, but introductions are hardest. Telling my birthplace is confusing. It has always seemed that I was born on another planet and snuck into Little Falls, New York, under a full moon, on August 19, 1948, Thursday.

I must come from the planet Newportia, by way of New York. Welcome to my world! Here, everything happens on time. People always mean what they say. You never have to do more than one thing at once. If you don't do it right at first, just try again. That is as Newportian as potato chip pie.

Everything necessary has been made and lasts forever. Since TV sets, radios and cars have only one channel, station or gear, that makes sense. The streets are paved with pizza. Edible clothes and furniture are the rage. When not raging.

Newportia has no crime. Giant parrots patrol my planet. They eat all criminal invaders. Our only work is feeding the parrots. Newportians bring bowls of fruit and popcorn to their beautiful friends. The popcorn comes from movie theaters. They feature two shows: Dumbo and Pinocchio.

Newportia usually is a postcard to me today. I can get along on Earth. Remember this: the reality and behavior of all autistics is just as sensible to them as your life. To ensure the fullest life possible for you and your children, you must accept them as human beings in every way.

Jerry Newport
Michigan

✦✦✦

121

"The Contributions of Sam"

I try to remind myself of all the things that Sam can do, and enjoys doing, instead of dwelling on all the "shortcomings." Of course, this is what I should do with all people. I try to stay hopeful about the future...the support that will be available in the schools, the home, the community that will enable Sam to become independent and productive. I also try to stay hopeful about the natural progress that Sam is going to continue to make, even though it is at a slow, unpredictable pace. I try to stay hopeful about my relationship with Sam...that even though he tests me a great deal, and can even be aggressive towards me, that I will find better ways to interact with him so that we can progress together as he matures.

SAM IS AN INTEGRAL PART OF THE RUSSELL FAMILY EXPERIENCE. We are who we are because he is a part of us. He is who he is because of the family he is in. I value this more than I can possibly communicate. Would I give away Sam's autism? Gladly! Would I give away the compassion and social awareness he has brought to my heart and the heart of my daughter, husband, and extended family and friends? Never! God has really used Sam to shape our lives, and I marvel at the strength of character, wisdom, and acceptance I see in my daughter...traits I never had at her young age, or will ever have in her natural, unfolding manner.

Anne Russell
Texas

◆◆◆

EPILOGUE

Several years ago, my daughter Jennifer was required to write a paper for her English class. She chose Alex as her subject. Until recently, I didn't know the paper existed. It only came to the surface as I was doing research for this book. It serves as a very appropriate epilogue to Laughing and Loving with Autism. *I'm sure you'll enjoy it.... almost as much as I did.*

Today I spoke with the only real Steppenwolf I know, only I had forgotten that I knew him. This person is my little brother, Alex. People think there is something very wrong with him because he can't (or won't) relate to other people. I see alot of him in me and am always surprised and a bit pleased whenever I become aware of these similarities. You see, I like to view my brother as being blessed rather than cursed. Alex was born with autism.

In case you are sitting there scratching your ear and wondering why that word sounds familiar, I will refresh your memory. Autism was the disorder that Dustin Hoffman had in *Rain Man*. Now, by no means did I grow up with a young Raymond Babbit. Alex can't do anything wonderful with numbers and he does not read phone books or count tooth picks. Yet he is cut off from most of the world.

That is about all I can say for certain. I do not know whether he was born away from us on the Mountain or if he has not even seen the fire that we think is light. I do not know this because he won't tell me. He does not write pages and pages filled with wise words. He does not paint emotional pictures. He does not compose music or make clay sculptures. I suppose he feels no need to vent his emotions. He only feels them.

You can read me anything that any scholar of autism has said to the contrary, but I am sure that Alex feels. He gets carried away by his emotion and forgets everything his parents have tried to teach him about how one should act in society. How can he restrain himself to society's rules if he isn't even aware of their presence?

He often skips absurdly around the house, stopping every once in a while to jump up and down in one spot while fixating on the ceiling. Usually while he is doing this, he is laughing. I don't know what he is laughing at. I guess it is just another of these things that he sees that we don't. I wish he would tell me what he is thinking, what he finds funny. Yet, he is still in his small upstairs room, and I don't even know if he has any desire to come out.

I said in the beginning of this paper that I saw much of Alex in me. I have always wondered if that made me somehow different from the rest of the world also. I usually don't like people to bother me. As a child, I would always upset my mother by closing myself in my room for hours on end. I never like to hear any noise from the outside world when I am trying to be alone. I was (and still am) forever shutting the door to my room, trying to close off the rest of the family, the T.V., and radios that are working in the house. I never understood why this upset my family. Alex was the first person to ever shut the door on *me*. He was the first person who ever told me to go away because he wanted to be alone. Though no one else understood that, I did.

Alex and I are also both very sensitive to sound. Any loud noise, even those that don't bother others will frighten us both. One recent example of this is when my father took us both to see a movie at a theater that both Alex and Dad, but not me, had been to. For the ten minutes before the movie started, Alex sat hunched over in his seat with his hands over his ears. Dad informed me that he was afraid of a buzzing sound that went off at that theater before the movie started. I knew that any sound that frightened him would probably also scare me, but as I look a lot like an adult type of person, I knew that I could not hunch over in my seat with my hands over my ears. Being the fool I am, I leaned over and teased my brother for being silly. I made myself forget about it and about two minutes later a buzzer went off. As my father loves to tell, I then yelped and jumped about a foot off my seat.

This sensitivity to noise also has its good sides. Both of us love music and will sit and listen to it for hours. I know he gets something out of the music he listens to because he always stops what he is doing and pays very close attention. His music is very important and must go undisturbed. Sometimes I forget this and start singing. Of course Alex is always there to kindly remind me to shut up.

Many times people (yes, even me) have tried to force my brother into getting out a piece of himself into the open for us to see. His answers are so trite and bizarre that I wonder if that is what he thinks or if he is making fun of the rest of us. Once when my father and Alex were driving through a piece of beautiful country with hills, trees and lakes, Dad asked Alex to turn to his right and tell what he saw. My brother looked in that direction, turned back to my father and answered, "A window."

When telling why I decided to change my story line, I gave the reason that I had recently spoken to Alex and realized that I must write about him. I did not speak with my brother over the phone, and since he does not live in this state (Texas, I mean. I'm not being philosophical, necessarily), I could not have spoken to him in person. I saw and conversed with Alex in a rather bizarre place, in a strange and vivid dream.

In this dream I found myself walking down the empty streets of my hometown, Baltimore. I seemed to be wandering but with feeling a sense of going somewhere. I turned a corner and saw a restaurant that had light coming from the window. It was bright, harsh light but it was light nonetheless, so I decided to investigate. The inside was almost as eerie as the streets outside. Everything was perfectly clean and orderly and the few people inside were silent. Normally, I would have passed by and kept to myself, but something about the place intrigued me. It seemed like the kind of place where anything was possible.

I ordered a cup of coffee and drifted into my own world as the man set the machine to make my hot bitter drink. Suddenly, I was startled as one of the men came and sat down beside me. For some reason, this seemed like the wrong place for conferring with others. In other restaurants it would have been strange, but somehow here it seemed unacceptable...and I liked it that way.

However, this man coming up to speak to me was not at all threatening, and his natural smile was comfortable and warm. He started to speak and his voice was familiar, but the words were not.

His face looked like I should know it somehow, but it was too...old? He kept on talking and for some reason I thought that he should not be using words so well, should not be speaking in such long, beautifully formed, eloquent sentences. Then, I felt a tremendous sense of joy as I realized who was sitting next to me and who was saying such wonderful things.

But, it couldn't be.

"Alex?"

He stopped his speech, "Yes?"

In the back of the restaurant I heard the beeping of the coffee machine.

Why wasn't the waiter going to turn it off?

Beep. Beep. Beep. Beep.

"This is wonderful, Alex. How did it happen? You can converse with me. You are finally part of our world!" For some reason there was an urgency to my speech, as if I had little time left.

And his last words came to me as I realized the beeping was the alarm and I was dreaming and had to get up.

"No, Jennifer, you have entered into my world."